GUT CONNECTION

A Coaches Guide to Anti-Inflammatory Living

GUT CONNECTION

A Coaches Guide to Anti-Inflammatory Living

A Taproots805 Production

Written By

ANNE E. FLETT

GUT
CONNECTION

A Coaches Guide to Anti-Inflammatory Living

Printed in the United States of America

Contents

The Framework

In a root system, the taproot grows the deepest.

It is the strongest.

It digs down into the depths and gathers and stores nourishment to support the entire root system.

Like the taproot, as individuals who desire a healthy environment in which to live, we must connect with and support others. It is essential that we take care of ourselves, spirit, mind and body, so that we can live our best lives and flow with nourishment and love for the people around us. To do this, we have to dig deep into our beliefs about ourselves. We must face the ugly side of ourselves and choose to love who we are and heal deeply, as no one else can do that for us. It is because the taproot digs deep that it can gather the nourishment it provides to the rest of the system.

Like a network of roots expanding the forested earth, we are all connected. Your energy, your mood, your attitude, and your actions have a ripple effect on the rest of society.

In a more direct sense, we are literally made of energy, vibrating, radiating, pulsating energy, which is constantly bumping up against, meshing with and bouncing off all the other energies around it.

We all matter.
We are all connected with one another.

In a world where children are being shot in school, violence is rampant and anger seems to rule so may, we need more than ever, to be healthy, to connect, to feel good and to love our lives so that we can then be good, loving and supportive to those around us.

There are opportunities for healing within connection.

Have you ever walked down the street, made eye contact with a stranger walking the opposite direction and felt a charge from the interaction? Or what about the opposite? You've been ready to make eye contact with the stranger, but they keep staring straight ahead or down at the ground leaving you without the brief moment of connection. There are times when just that quick exchange made when making eye contact can make a difference in a person's day. Just the acknowledgement of not being alone, the acknowledgement of being seen, can shift an attitude. It seems so minute but is so important.

When we don't feel good, when we are dealing with pain, extra weight, health conditions, or if we are caught in our heads, replaying scenarios that we have no power to change, again and again, we are unable to connect and nourish those around us. When we are feeling powerless to change, or guilty because we want to do one thing yet find ourselves doing another, or we have a pattern we would like to change, yet never seem to be able to, our ability to be a positive force in the life of those we love is diminished.

This book is about ridding your body of inflammation, but at its core, it's truly about connection. The answer to all of this hurt, I believe is to be found there. It's in being able to look someone in the eye and authentically connect with them. It's about understanding that you, by taking care of yourself, are making this world a better place. When you feel good, when your body feels good, when you feel confident and strong, you are more likely to make others feel good. On the flip side, when you are angry or feeling inferior, you are more likely to spread anger or behave like a jerk.

My true desire is to help you be like the taproot.

In my years as a personal trainer, I have spoken with people every day who were in pain or trying to manage some condition or ailment, most of which were associated with inflammation. I began coaching people on an anti-inflammatory lifestyle, how to rid their body of chronic inflammation, how to heal their gut and detoxify their homes as well as their thoughts. The physical relief that comes with the elimination of the pain, puffiness and weariness associated with chronic inflammation is transformative!

My intention here is to help you move into a lifestyle which is proven to be preventative of disease and healthy for your spirit, mind and body. This is not a strict diet where you will be measuring your food and counting your calories. Rather, it is intended to be sustainable from the very beginning. It's a lifestyle change rather than a diet, and it's centered on gratitude and gut health.

SO....

For a moment, stop and consider your body.
Feel your lungs as they fill with air.
Feel your heart beating in your chest.
Listen.
Feel the energy around you.

As your lungs fill feel the wave of oxygen move through your body.

Our bodies are incredible!
What mechanics!
What chemistry!
How completely intricate!

Marvel with me for a moment here.

Consider the environment.
The animals
The food chains
The ecosystems

The Sun!

...in its perfect spacing and positioning!

The weather!

Trees!

Have you read The_Hidden Life of Trees?!

It will forever change your view of our forests, plants and trees.

Consider food.

Consider how it grows out of the earth

...to nourish us

We may have amazing food that comes out of packages but there is nothing that is going to change the fact that we are natural, organic beings in an amazing world, that when studied, never fails to fascinate. We may separate ourselves from the natural world through pavement, buildings, fancy cars, movies, and the like, but we'll always be a part of it. We are connected to the natural world on the most organic level and to think ourselves separate from it is as futile as it is damaging to our spirits, our minds, and our bodies.

Like the rhythm of our hearts, so too our lives have a rhythm, our energy has a rhythm, our days have rhythm. To live our very best lives, to be in tune to the rhythm around us, healthy, pain free and to have vitality, means nourishing ourselves on food that grows from the earth. It means connecting with the source of it all, in whatever way you choose to define or not define it, through spirit, mind and body.

Consider our minds.
Our brains.
Our emotions.
The unseen factors that shape our realities.

Consider spirituality.
Faith.

I ask you to marvel with me at how amazing all of this is!

I ask you to do this because I want you to be ramped up for success in transitioning to an anti-inflammatory lifestyle.

At the heart of all that you do,

at the center of everything,

there MUST be gratitude.

And I don't mean a shopping list of things in your life you are thankful for, kind of gratitude. I mean "Oh my gosh, I can't handle the wonder of it all!", kind of gratitude. I mean AWE!

More than gratitude, the real gem at the center of it all is wonder, amazement, and AWE, at how INCREDIBLE this whole world is.

Become fascinated.

Connect, emotionally with the wonder of it all.

Recognize how incredible this whole world and the life it contains is. Your body is a fascinating part of it. Like a chemistry set, it will respond to what you put into it. I speak of more than just food when I say that, by the way, what you feed your mind through media and interests pursued, the conversations and thoughts that fill your day is paramount to your overall success. Equally important is that you feed and tend to your spirit. My hope is that achieving balance in your gut will lead or add to finding balance in all areas of your life.

Gratitude is the gem for several reasons. One is when you have gratitude, wonder and awe you will find more things to have gratitude, wonder and awe about. Your focus will shift toward those things and the Law of Attraction will bring you even more to find. Whatever you focus on in life, you will get more of. What do you want more of?

Practicing gratitude for the natural world will make it easier to choose to chomp on broccoli and blueberries because you'll appreciate how miraculous food and its healing power is. A division from packaged, processed, convenience and sugar filled foods on an emotional level is much more powerful than just practicing willpower by saying "no". Willpower has its place but being entirely not interested is even better. Gratitude for what is grown from the Earth to nourish you and gratitude for your body will help you get to there.

Gratitude will help you to be happier each day.

When it comes to lifestyle change, our thoughts, beliefs and mindset are half the battle which is why the second part of this book is dedicated to them. Truly, we all know how we SHOULD eat. We all know we SHOULD workout, but actually doing them can become a huge stumbling block. Have you ever wondered why?

Let's dig deep. Let's examine your deeply held beliefs about yourself and your health. Let's examine the words you nourish yourself with.

The best possible thing we can do is live our best lives, nurturing our spirits, minds, and bodies so that we can better connect with and love those around us. Taking care of yourself in this way, nourishing your body and ridding it of inflammation is a powerful source of self-love and wellness. You not only make yourself healthier, but with your success and through this practice, you can better support and love those around you. Your energy is bound to increase, and you will marvel at how your body will react to this change.

Changing my nutrition not only took away my pain, decreased my weight, increased my energy, and improved my skin, but it also empowered me to take more control in all areas of my life. I began living in a proactive way regarding my health, rather than in a reactionary way that would have me on prescription drugs and under a surgeon's knife (without a discussion on nutrition to be had). It wasn't long after that I began shaping my reality in other areas of life rather than living in a reactionary, non-empowered way. For me, success in nutrition led to success in all other areas. Changing my diet changed my life and I am happier, more energetic, leaner and stronger in spirit, mind and body, than I was before. Oh yeah, I'm in a lot less pain too.

There is only one you; and you are necessary.

No one else has your make up of gifts, talents, strengths and experiences. No one else has your same perspectives or can shine the way you can shine in this world. Loving yourself enough to make this change will allow you to flourish and thrive. You can focus on other areas of your life because your pain and inflammation will no longer be in your way. You will be better able to love and connect with others. Your focus will improve.

It takes courage to live life to its fullest. I hope you are living the life you have seen for yourself for so long. I hope you are doing something that lights you up, fills you. I know that ridding your body of inflammation is only going to make you stronger and better and I'm excited for your journey.

You want to feel good and to rock this life that you have!

You do not have to be in chronic pain!

You don't want to be uncomfortable in your own skin.

You are the only you that this planet has

....and we would be deprived of your full brilliance if you let it be diminished by something you could control and the pain that goes with it.

Inflammation is at the heart of most diseases: heart disease, diabetes, cancer, arthritis, neurological disease, autoimmune disease, and fatty liver disease are just a few. It plays a role in your allergies, asthma, depression, joint pain, Alzheimer's, and IBS. By gaining control of your diet you can eliminate inflammation and regain the health and vitality you know is possible.

My Story

It's interesting that if I look at some of the most major decisions, I've made in life I can distinctly remember having strong resistance to that choice before coming around to choose it. For instance, I didn't want to go to San Diego State University because so many people in my area chose to go there, and yet it is where I went. I didn't want to consider becoming a teacher, I never wanted to move to Santa Barbara, and I hated my health classes in school. Check, check, check! It's almost the greater goodness that decision is going to bring me, the greater my resistance is to it. In that light, it makes total sense that I am passionate about sharing what I have learned about managing my health through nutrition, supplementing, mindset and a healthy lifestyle.

Our mind body connection is powerful. The words we speak over ourselves and where we place our focus determine our outcome. There have been many things over the past decade that have made me marvel at our bodies. We are so intricately amazing! We are like these wonderful chemistry sets that respond to what we feed them; spirit, mind and body. The occurrence that changed my life, the one that tipped the scales permanently in favor of complete wellness, however, was discovering that I was bone on bone in my left hip.

When you are in pain, real pain day after day, it can be difficult to ignore. It can become difficult to be nice and it can prevent you from doing things you would normally do. About 7 years ago I began to notice that when I stood up from being seated, I would somewhat hobble around until my hip kicked into action. Soon I noticed pain radiating from around my hip, the pain eventually would make its way from my hip to my toes. Night after night I was in pain from my hip to my toes. I could feel my bones and they hurt. It felt good, like a little massage, to hit my hip gently. Not long after that, I noticed marked weakness on my left side. If I were going up stairs, I'd need to lead with my right leg, not my left because it was too weak to support the step up. My range of motion was affected and soon I could no longer sit crossed legged on the floor nor cross my left ankle over my right knee. In bed at night, I could not lay on my right side as the weight of my left hip would pull downward, causing pain. If I kept my phone in my back pocket for too long the weight of it would cause pain in my hip. Does any of this sound familiar or hold true to what you have experienced?

When my doctor told me that I'd be a candidate for a hip replacement, I was in total shock. Although I've always been athletic, it was far from what my water retaining, baby weight carrying, completely inflamed self, identified as. Plus, I was a swimmer! My non-impact sport should have been kind to my joints, but heredity, nutrition and my need for action dictated something else.

When the doctor told me, they were going to put me on anti-inflammatory drugs, I drew the line. I am far too much of a natural child to go on prescription drugs without trying alternate methods first. I called up Sonia, my in-family expert, and we discussed inflammation. Sonia is an ostomy nurse who also happens to be an esthetician. She is a specialist on healing, intestinal care, skin and nutrition who also fully embraces holistic, integrated medicine, Eastern medicine and supplementing. She is reiki trained. She led me to some good sources, and I absorbed it all.

I changed my diet to a highly anti-inflammatory one and learned all I could about managing inflammation and pain. Nutrition is the major component but strengthening and mindset are also vital.

Within 2 weeks of my diet change I began to notice a reduction in my pain. By about a month in, my pain was almost completely gone and so were at least five of my extra pounds! The beautiful side effect to eating to reduce pain is that you are also eating for a healthy life! Extra pounds melt off of your body and your energy level greatly increases. There is really no need for outside motivation or help once you really get the hang of the anti-inflammatory diet, the way you will feel is motivation in itself.

A few years ago, I began experimenting with running on the beach and on the trails. Would you believe it is a non-issue! I run 7 miles with ease about 3 times a week, but only on the sand and trails, never on the pavement. The same doctor who told me not to run or walk for exercise anymore is absolutely impressed. He has declared that beyond eliminating the pain, I am actually repairing the hip through self-care.

I cannot say that everyone will have my results. I can only coach you along your journey, but it is something I really want to do. If I can help you overcome your pain or even just transition to a very healthy proactive way of eating regardless of if you have pain or not, I want to do it. Our health is too important, and we need it to rock this life we have!

Speaking of change, gaining control of your diet, your weight, your health, is SO EMPOWERING! It was because of this change in my life that I have had the courage and the vision to make the sweeping changes that I have made in recent years. It's because of this that I know that I am in control of my life and am no longer living in a reactionary manner. Beside the fact that I lost over twenty pounds and have kept it off with ease, my skin and eyes are clear, and my energy is abundant, I am living pain free, I am perfectly healthy and I feel amazing!

What is Inflammation

Most kids on the playground are familiar with classic acute inflammation. A trip, and fall resulting in scraped knees or abraded hands will also induce acute inflammation. It's part of the body's inflammatory response, where our body increases production of white blood cells, immune cells and substances called cytokines that help fight infection. Classic signs of acute inflammation include redness, pain, heat and swelling. As the wound heals, the swelling subsides, and your body has once again reacted in it's amazing and perfect way! Insert great expressions of gratitude here that our bodies are so amazing!

On the other hand, chronic inflammation is often silent, and occurs inside the body often without any noticeable symptoms. Many people live for years or even nearly a lifetime with chronic inflammation damaging their organs silently. This chronic inflammation can drive conditions like diabetes, heart disease, fatty liver disease, asthma, eczema, neurological disorders, irritable bowel syndrome, arthritis and cancer.

Inflammation in itself is symptomatic of larger issues. On its own, it is only a symptom for which your doctor may test to find the root problem. Chronic inflammation is always indicative of a health issue which must be addressed. If you are battling chronic inflammation, you must work with your health practitioner to find the cause of it. Additionally, ridding your body of chronic inflammation will not only make you feel better, increase your energy and vitality, but it will also pave a clear and nutrient filled road to healing. Inflammation tests may include markers for C-reactive protein (CRP), homocysteine, TNF alpha and IL-6. (4)

Exposure to the toxins in our cleansers, carpets, containers, car emissions and so many other sources play a role in chronic inflammation. Always protect yourself against unnecessary toxin exposure by wearing a mask if you are using any chemical laden product such as paint or resin. Avoid heavy, industrial cleansers. There are many natural products available in even the mainstream grocery stores that a switch would be easy and beneficial to your health. Furthermore, as our awareness of toxins in cleansers has become clearer there have been some fantastic alternative products developed. Norwex is a Norwegian company that produces microfiber cloths which require no cleansers, just water, to remove 99% of bacteria. With a little research, you can find many toxin free options for your home. Plus, there's always good, old fashioned apple cider vinegar with water. Which really is a fantastic option. Killing 98% of germs and also healthy to digest, cleansing your system, apple cider vinegar sure beats bleach which kills 99% of germs but is toxic. (46)

Choosing to buy organic rather than chemical sprayed foods is a major component to eliminating ingested toxins.

One major source of inflammation is our American diet. Rich in "Healthy Whole Wheat", factory farmed & processed meat, it is sugar laden with a healthy serving of fast food, MSG, sodium on the side, a soda to go with it and it will also lead to chronic inflammation. Built on a mixture of convenience, greed, science and a desire to feed the masses our current mainstream food options are far from being sourced from the earth and far from truly nourishing our bodies. The next time you are opening a package of food, ask yourself whether it is adding to the inflammation in your body, or taking away the inflammation. Make this a habit.

Toxins absorbed through our skin, breathed in, ingested in our food, or any other means, contribute considerably to a condition called Leaky Gut, which leads many to chronic inflammation and to a road that leads to organ destruction.

In fact, all health is rooted in the gut. It is essential to keep our guts in balance, to avoid the pendulum swing from diarrhea to constipation, to balance our hormones, and to have a rock-solid foundation from which to absorb nutrients and live a healthy life.

It's All About the Gut

That's right. When it comes down to it, all health is largely centered in our intestines. In fact, over two thirds of your immune system are garrisoned there. (32) Research has found that there are over 40 trillion bacteria cells in your body, compared to 30 trillion human cells. (33) (34) Although some reside on our skin and in our mouths, most of these bacteria, along with viruses, fungi and other microorganisms, reside in your intestines, specifically in your large intestine. The gut "microbiome", as it is referred to is extremely important to your health. When put together the microbiome weighs 2-5 pounds (1-2 kg), which is roughly the weight of the human brain. (35)

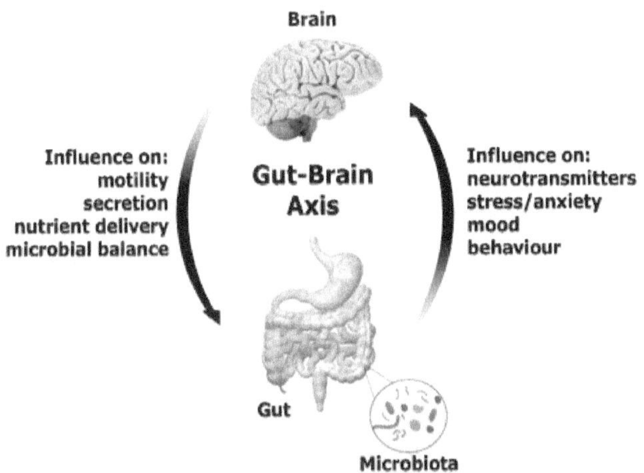

Holistic practitioners, for years, have called our gut the "third brain" and have talked about our mind body connection and how powerful it is. Now in Western medicine, as more research is done and more facts about our microbiome are coming to light, it is largely agreed upon that our gut is like a third brain. Controlling more than our digestion, it is closely tied to our mental health. The health of your microbiome will affect more than your absorption of minerals, and defenses against toxins and inflammation. It will affect your mood swings, anxiety levels, stress levels, clarity of thinking and general outlook on life.

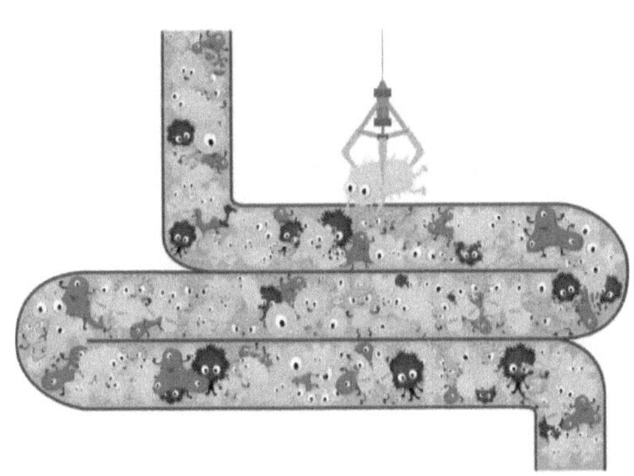

Credit: Yang H. Ku/Shutterstock/C&ENt

The bacteria in our bodies can be both "good" and "bad". ([36]) It's okay that there is a small percentage of "bad" bacteria in our systems, the idea is to not let them thrive and grow. For instance, we all have some e-coli bacteria nesting in our intestines but if that particular bacteria were to multiply and thrive you would become extremely ill. Nourishing your body with natural, anti-inflammatory foods will keep your microbiome in a healthy balance. Your immune system will strengthen, your inflammation will decrease and so will your pain, skin conditions, gas problems and so on.

We want to keep a healthy balance of bacteria so that there are plenty of good bacteria which provide for so many functions in our bodies, and to keep the number of bad bacteria low. Probiotic foods, such as fermented foods, miso, tempeh, and acidophilus containing yogurt and kefirs add good bacteria into your system, as do probiotic supplements. Other foods, known as prebiotics feed the good bacteria promoting its health and yours. Onion, garlic, leeks, asparagus and apples are just a few of these gut friendly, prebiotic foods.

These foods are especially important if you are on antibiotics which kill good bacteria in your intestines.

Leaky Gut

Often Leaky Gut is at the root of our inflammation. There are a certain number of you who do not have major disease or massive amounts of joint pain, you simply have Leaky Gut due to lifestyle factors and nutrition. In either case, tightening and repairing the gut and ridding our bodies of chronic inflammation are our main objectives.

Symptoms of Leaky Gut are:

- Gas and bloating and cramping, Irritable Bowel Syndrome
- Headaches
- Food sensitivities
- Brain fog
- Nutritional deficiencies
- Excessive or chronic fatigue, fibromyalgia
- Joint pain
- Skin conditions such as eczema, rosacea, rashes, acne and psoriasis.
- Depression, anxiety, ADD or ADHD
- Autoimmune disease

Does anybody really like the term Leaky Gut?

Gross right?

The term is spot on however, and if we can defend our gut walls by taking away the inflammation, making them nice and secure against the toxins that would otherwise invade our bloodstream, we can prevent most illnesses. Let me say that again. By taking care of our gut lining, we can keep toxins out of our bloodstream and prevent most illnesses.

What?! By keeping toxins and unnatural things out of our bloodstream we can prevent most illnesses? You mean, living closer to nature and eating the food provided for us by this planet and the sun revolving around it in perfect positioning, is the key to being healthy!? ... Seriously, if you wrap your heart and mind around this concept while also being full of gratitude for it, it will make you want to eat only natural foods. Why would we even want something processed and packaged?

Revel in our connection to the Earth, eat from it, embrace what is natural reject what is not natural and heal your own gut connection in the process.

While it's true that digestion begins in the mouth then stomach, most digestion and absorption of nutrients occurs in the intestines, which also work to defend against foreign invaders like pathogens and toxins. When inflammation causes a weak spot in the wall, a leak, the pathogens and toxins slip into the bloodstream causing white blood cells to swarm in and do their job of attacking the invaders. Too often however, the excess of white blood cells working hard cause healthy organs to be attacked. An example per the American Heart Association is that when chronic inflammation stays too long in blood vessels it promotes the buildup of plaque which is then perceived as a foreign invader. It tries to wall off the plaque from blood flow inside the arteries which can become unstable and rupture leading to blood clotting, blocking the flow of blood to the heart or brain resulting in stroke or heart attack. (61) Chronic inflammation can lead to DNA damage which results in some forms of cancer. (61)

When functioning correctly, the cells that line the intestines, called the mucosa, are linked securely together with tight junction proteins that create a barrier and regulate the substances that pass into your bloodstream. While vital nutrients are let through; foreign substances such as toxins, microbes, and certain food components are mostly kept out. Those that do slip through are swiftly tagged by the immune system with antibodies to signal white blood cells to get rid of them. Again, this is a wonderful place to express gratitude at how amazing our bodies are!

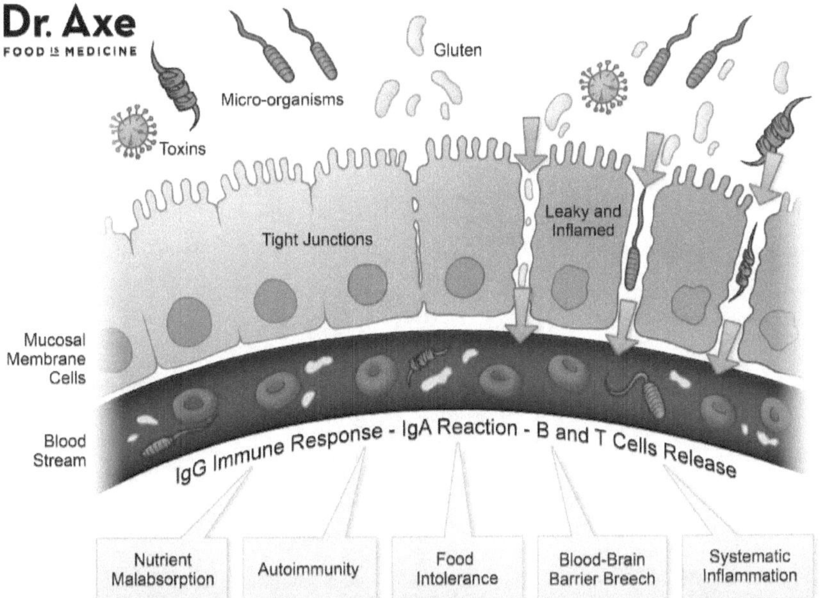

However, if an irregularity occurs in the mucosal cells and the integrity of the protective barrier weakens, gaps and holes may develop, increasing intestinal permeability, according to a study in the journal Frontiers in Immunology. Once the intestinal lining has been compromised, undigested foreign proteins, including food components not broken down by normal digestion, "leak" into the bloodstream in high concentrations. This is what's commonly referred to as leaky gut. (1)

The foreign substances that overwhelm the immune system, create an inflammatory response that leads to problems in the digestive tract and throughout the entire body. Ultimately, a leaky gut has the potential to affect more than your bowels. High levels of white blood cells are needed to do their job, they attack healthy organs, and can set the stage for a long list of systemic problems. (1)

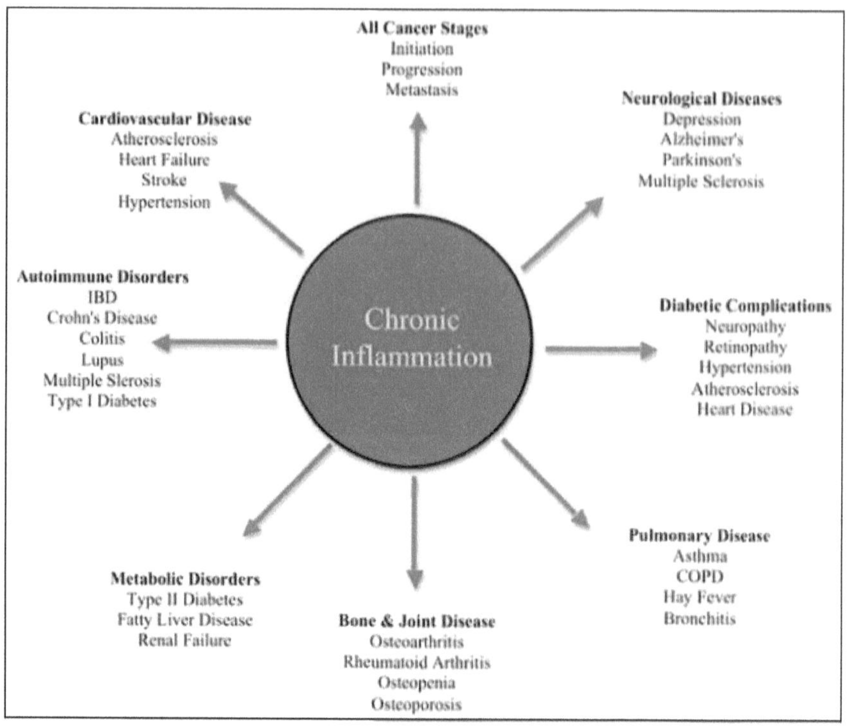

Image borrowed from Cedar Mountain Herb School

Your gut health is foundational to your overall wellness. It is the cornerstone upon which your health is built. Eliminating inflammation, tightening your gut walls and restoring good flora and fauna will transform your health. Our bodies are intricate chemistry sets and what we put in them really does matter. You will lose weight; your pain will go away and your energy and vitality will increase!

Causes of Leaky Gut include:

- Sugar
- Use of NSAID's
- Alcohol

- Nutrient deficiencies
- Inflammation
- Stress
- Poor gut health
- Yeast overgrowth
- Environmental toxins

While the mainstream medical community has yet to confirm Leaky Gut Syndrome as a root cause for many of today's diseases, evidence is mounting that it is at the source. In fact, according to Harvard Medical School; "There may never be such a single path, mounting evidence suggests a common underlying cause of major degenerative diseases. The four horsemen of the medical apocalypse — coronary artery disease, diabetes, cancer, and Alzheimer's — may be riding the same steed: inflammation." (62)

Let's Talk About Wheat

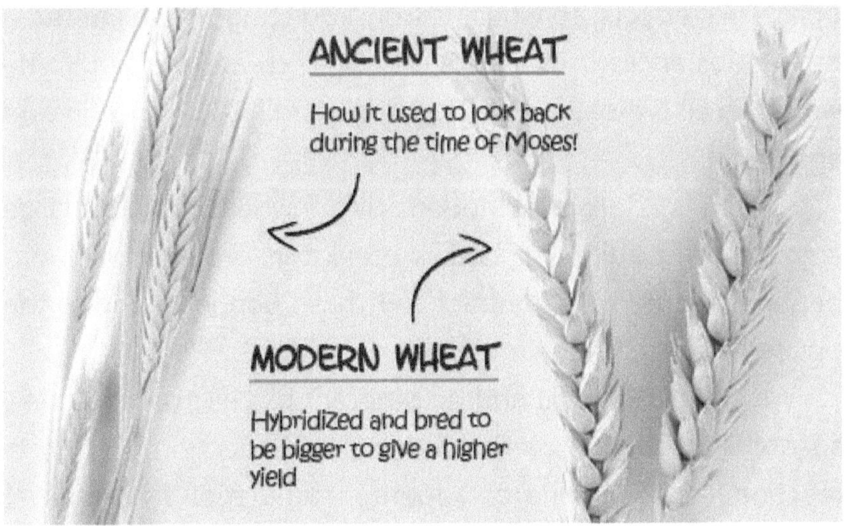

Conventional nutrition would have you include healthy whole wheat bread in your day to day diet. The fact is that wheat, long held as a staple in our diet, has been modified to the point that our bodies can no longer process it efficiently. (3)

In the 1960's, in order to yield more crops for less money, dwarf wheat was created. The benefits of a high-yield crop are obvious, but it comes at a price. Specifically, modern wheat has some subtle but important differences in its nutrient and protein composition which weakens our gut linings. (4)

With reduced zinc, iron, magnesium and copper concentrations, there are more problematic strains of gluten proteins in modern wheat which our bodies cannot process, particularly in those with celiac or severe gluten sensitivities. This causes intestinal permeability, also known as Leaky Gut Syndrome. (5)

Modern Dwarf Wheat contains the gliadin protein which acts as appetite stimulant. Do you find yourself reaching for another cracker, another dose of wheat, several times a day? According to Dr. Davis, author of <u>Wheat Belly</u>, the gliadin protein has opiate-like effects, so wheat is truly addicting. There are three other substances in wheat that help to create the syndrome we now call "wheat belly": They are gliadin, amylopectin and agglutinin. (4)

Gliadin is a protein. Modern dwarf wheat contains large amounts of gliadin. Our bodies break this protein down into peptides in the digestive tract and those peptides bind to the opiate receptors in the brain. (4)

We are all different and on different places in our journey, so not all people experience the same reaction. Common reactions to gliadin are: appetite stimulation, withdrawal symptoms that come about two hours after eating wheat and wheat products, and dependency. In short, gliadin creates an addiction to wheat. Wheat is not a food to just cut back on. Eating less wheat will not get rid of the problem. You will still be addicted and craving more. Wheat must be eliminated from your diet entirely.

Amylopectin is a carbohydrate contained in wheat. The blood sugar high from eating wheat is often followed by sudden crashes, which happen over about a two-hour cycle. This is why so many people go through a cycle of eating foods high in sugar and flour, then crashing two hours later, experiencing brain fog, headaches and other symptoms, then craving more. (6)

Food companies love it, and put it in virtually everything, from soup to salad dressing and even licorice: the more you eat, the more you crave. It's addicting, convenient and inexpensive and as a result, you buy more food. (6)

Lastly, there is agglutinin. Agglutinin is found in the germ of the wheat and is thought to interfere with the production and release of leptin, the hormone that signals fullness or satiety. (6)

When combined with amylopectin and glutenin, you have a vicious trio: together, they trigger a dependency on foods high in sugar and flour, plus an inability to tell when you are satisfied. Is one doughnut ever really enough? (6)

The addiction to high calorie foods and inability to recognize when to stop eating them is a huge factor to all of that excess visceral fat around the abdomen. It's also responsible for chronic inflammation, type 2 diabetes, heart disease and other issues related to obesity, skin conditions and the host of other ailments that go along with the inflammation. Unfortunately, this has been normalized in society and is a way of life for many.

It is essential for optimal health and in order to thrive on this amazing, wild, organic planet, to connect with what your body is telling you and to choose to take care of it.

As long as you consume wheat, you are not in control over your impulses, appetite or inflammation. (3) While eliminating it from your diet seems daunting, it might be easier than you think. If you are prepared ahead of time with other food options and ready to grab snacks, it makes the change much easier. After two weeks without wheat you should begin to feel the difference in your body and that will encourage you further. Plus, by eliminating wheat entirely you eliminate the strong cravings and addiction, ultimately making your journey much easier.

When you eliminate wheat, you may experience withdrawal effects. I therefore recommend eliminating it in stages.

1.   Get rid of the biggest offenders

The biggies include bread, pasta, breaded foods, pastries and crackers.

2.   Stop consuming packaged foods that contain wheat

...such as breaded chicken or fish sticks, cereals, packaged snack foods.

3.   Prepare yourself by having the right foods on hand

The easiest way to fall off the bandwagon is by not having the right choices nearby when you are hungry and need sustenance right away. Before you dive into the gluten-free pool, be sure to stock up on food that you love that is also gluten-free. Trek Mix is something I always have on hand in case of an emergency. For others, carrying a piece of fruit or a nutritious bar does the trick.

4.   Become a wheat sleuth

...by uncovering and avoiding hidden wheat by reading ingredients. Refrain from buying dressings, sauces and seasonings that contain wheat.

5.   Focus on what you can eat!

This is major!!!

Where you place your focus truly determines your success. If you focus on what you can't eat, you'll be thinking about those foods and solidifying a negative attitude about a lifestyle from which you will gain so much. Instead, focus on what you can eat and connect with a sense of wonder and gratitude that it was sourced from this amazing Earth, made perfectly to run your body, and is actually improving your health.

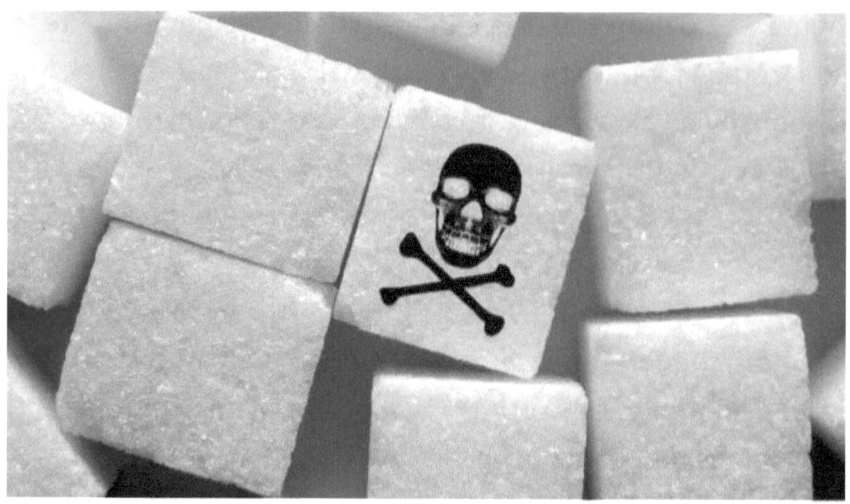

Thank you BBC for the picture

What about Sugar?

It's commonly known that sugar is toxic to our bodies and that the American diet is full of hidden sugars. When you begin to pay attention to food labels you will be shocked by how much sugar is in packaged and processed foods. You will find it in your sauces, dressings, seasoning packets, breaded foods, chips as well as the dip you are dipping them in. Why is it in so much? Well, it's addicting, that's why.

While the recommended daily allowance of sugar for women is 6 teaspoons a day, and for men 9 teaspoons, according to the Center for Disease Control the average American consumes an average of 19.5 teaspoons a day. Wow! According to the US National Institute on Drug abuse, sugar is addicting and can affect the brain much like cocaine or alcohol does.

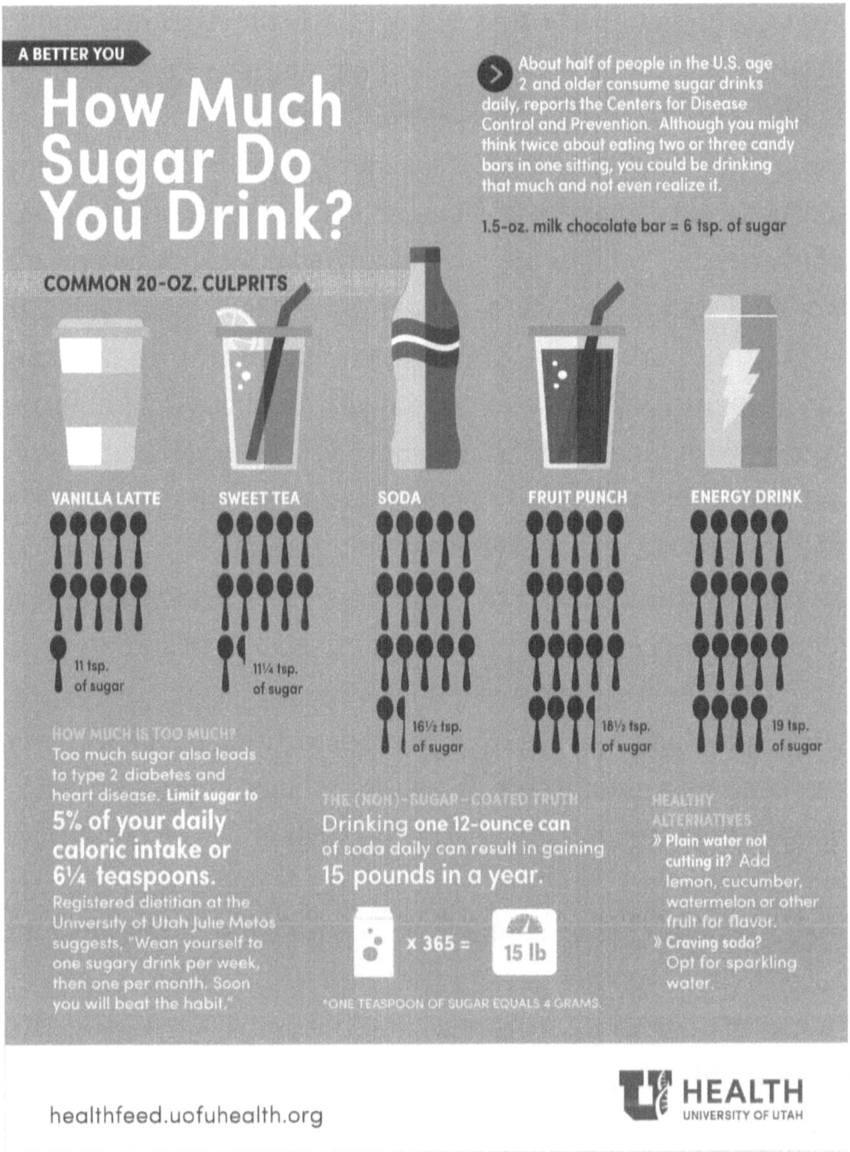

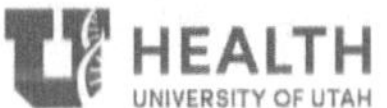

According to The Center For Disease Control, sweetened beverages are a leading source of increased sugar consumption leading to weight gain/obesity, type 2 diabetes, heart disease, kidney diseases, non-alcoholic liver disease, tooth decay and cavities, as well as gout. Soda, energy drinks, sweetened coffee drinks and juice are beverages consumed without much thought given to the outstanding amount of sugars they are made with. According to Livestrong.com, a 12 ounce can of Coke contains 39 grams of total sugar. Do you know how many teaspoons of sugar that is? No, I can't convert that off of the top of my head either and the food industry knows it. It's a brilliant way to disguise the fact that there are 9.3 teaspoons of sugar in that one can. The recommended daily allowance of sugar for women is 6 teaspoons per day. For men, it's 9. No matter your gender, one can of soda exceeds your daily limit. If you are a soda drinker, chances are you drink more than one in a day and this alone is adversely affecting your health. According to WomensHealth.com drinking 1 to 2 cans of soda a day will increase your chance of getting type 2 diabetes by 26%.

Fruit juice may seem like a healthy alternative, but in the large quantities we are accustomed to drinking them, they can become a sugar snare. If we served juice in the small juice glasses of yesteryear, it may not be such an issue, but as it is we do everything large in this country. Coupled with the fact that one glass of juice contains several pieces of fruits worth of juice, it's as if you are getting the sugar from several pieces of fruit with none of the fiber that the fruit actually contains. The fiber found in a whole piece of fruit is vital as it slows down the process of sugars going into your liver. If you drink a glass of fruit juice which has no fiber, however, the sugars are sent quickly to you liver causing it to metabolize the juice much like it would a can of soda, poorly. (55) The high levels of fructose sugar can store as fat and do lead to insulin resistance. If you are diabetic or obese, this can complicate an already unhealthy situation.

12 oz. of Coca Cola contains 140 calories and 40 grams (10 teaspoons) of sugar.

12 oz. of juice contains 165 calories and 39 (9.8 teaspoons) of sugar. (55)

According to a recent article published on CNN.com (56), in a study where individuals drank more than 10% of their daily caloric intake in sugary beverages, they had a 44% higher chance of dying from cardiovascular disease and a 14% higher chance of dying from any other cause, than those who drank under 5% of their intake in sugary beverages.

We were not made to consume sugar at this rate. If we are thinking along the lines of living closer to the Earth, to the natural and the organic because it is vital to our success as living beings, we must drastically reduce our sugar intake. Sugar is directly linked to diabetes, weight gain, heart disease, cancer, fatty liver, depression, acne and more.

As an alternate to the sugar-rich sodas, coffee drinks, energy drinks and juices, you might try mineral water with a splash of cranberry juice or kombucha which will aid your gut health. Green tea or matcha are both excellent energizers and juice replacers. Water infused with mint, cucumber, berries, ginger, or citrus is always refreshing.

All of these are sugar:

Agave Sugar	Diastase	Panocha
Blackstrap	Fructose	Sorghum Syrup
molasses	Glucose	Turbinado Sugar
Cane Sugar	Grape Sugar	Beet Sugar
Confectioners	Invert Sugar	Cane Juice Crystals
Sugar	Maltose	Castor Sugar
Date Sugar	Organic Raw Sugar	Crystalline
Diastatic malt	Rice Syrup	Fructose
Florida Crystals	Treacle	Dextrose
Galactose	Barley Malt	Evaporated Cane
Golden Syrup	Buttered Syrup	Juice
Icing Sugar	Carob Syrup	Fruit Juice
Maltodextrin	Corn Syrup Solids	Concentrate
Muscovado	Dextran	Golden Sugar
Refiner's Sugar	Ethyl Maltol	Honey
Sugar	Fruit Juice	Malt Syrup
Barbados Sugar	Glucose Solids	Molasses
Brown Sugar	High Fructose	Raw Sugar
Carmel	Corn Syrup	Sucrose
Corn Syrup	Lactose	Yellow Sugar
Demerara Sugar	Maple Syrup	

Breaking the sugar addiction is essential in an anti-inflammatory lifestyle, however, a sudden break from the sugar addiction can cause withdrawal symptoms such as headaches, fatigue, depression and achiness. Therefore, I recommend eliminating sugar in stages.

1.   Decide what you are counting as sugar

For some no sugar means giving up sugary foods such as candy, pastries and soda. Others may be ready to go a step further and eliminate sugar from fruit, dried fruit and natural sweeteners such as honey or maple syrup. Set your boundaries.

2.   Prepare yourself by having the right foods on hand

The easiest way to fall off the bandwagon is by not having the right choices nearby when you are hungry and need sustenance right away. Before you dive into the sugar-free (or gluten-free) pool, be sure to stock up on food that you love that is also sugar-free. Trek Mix is something I always have on hand in case of an emergency. For others, carrying a piece of fruit or a nutritious bar does the trick.

3.   Eliminate the biggies

Soda, sweet coffee drinks, energy drinks, desserts, ultra-processed snack foods, and sugar cereals are among the biggest offenders. In the first week, stick with eliminating these big guys. It'll only take 2 weeks for your body to adjust to the new normal.

4.   Eliminate the sneaky ones

Folks, sugar is everywhere. In your second week of eliminating sugar from your diet, go ahead and start reading labels. Your salad dressing. Full of sugar? Don't forget to look at the sauces, soy, teriyaki, BBQ, all loaded with sugar. Go ahead and ponder why it is that we got so far from natural and consider what it is that you truly want for your body. I doubt being bombarded with sugars is your answer.

Don't forget to live!
A sugar-free diet is admirable, but it's okay to celebrate your nephew's birthday with the occasional piece of cake. Remember, this is meant to add to your quality of life, not to dampen it down.

Assignment:

What are 3 changes you can make today to reduce the amount of sugar you consume?
1.

2.

3.

Dare We Talk About Dairy?

Dairy is a mixed bag of love and inflammation for most. Approximately 65% of all Americans are lactose intolerant .(48) What's distressing,(especially for those standing downwind), is that many don't realize that their gas, bloating, abdominal pain and pendulum swing from diarrhea to constipation are due to dairy. So, many people continue to eat a diet heavy with dairy; cereal with cow's milk in the morning, half and half in their coffee, yogurt midday, a salad with ranch dressing and shredded cheese at lunch, a burger with cheese for dinner followed by ice cream before bed.

Whether it's a true lactose intolerance, where your body does not produce the lactase enzyme needed to break down the lactose, as sugar found in milk, or a lactose sensitivity the inflammatory response created by it can be devastating to your health. When your gut is inflamed your immunity is down and your healthy organs are in distress. Additionally, that inflamed gut could lead to more toxins entering your bloodstream causing even more system wide inflammation leading to illness and disease.

Our obsession with cow's milk products is entirely man made and driven by the fact that cows are the easiest of the beasts to milk with a high yield of milk. Excellent as an additional source of nutrition for early pastoral community's milk thrives under the false pretenses that today also, it is a necessary addition to our diets. It's not. Just as we no longer need our human mothers' milk now that we are no longer infants, our communities (in most places), have grown and we now have widespread access to nutrition and do not have to be reliant on milk to fill the gaps.

Thank you, Mind Body Green, for the following list!

10 Excellent, Non-Dairy, sources of calcium:
    Almonds
    Kale
    Oranges
    Collard Greens
    Broccoli
    Figs
    Spinach
    Enriched rice, almond, hemp and coconut milks
    Sesame seeds
    Tofu

Things to Consider

Changing your diet and ridding your body of inflammation is one of the most healthy and proactive decisions you could make. Congratulations on the choice to truly care for yourself on this level!

We are all in different places regarding our health and the issues surrounding chronic inflammation. There is, most likely, emotion, heartache, physical pain, and a real journey surrounding your arrival to this place. This is a real lifestyle change if you are ready for it to be, because this change feels so good you may become obsessed with the power of good nutrition!

Consider how you want to begin the new way of eating.

Some may choose to fast before starting. There are many health benefits to fasting. In short, without putting energy towards digestion, your body has more energy to put towards restoring other things. A fresh and rested gut is a great starting point for this dietary change.

Others who may or may not fast, choose to do a detox before beginning the new way of eating. A detox basically means cleansing the blood. This is done by removing impurities from the blood in the liver, where toxins are processed for elimination. While it is true that our bodies detoxify themselves daily, if you have a buildup of processed and sugar laden, westernized foods in your system the additional, intentional detox will be beneficial. If you are under the care of a physician, discuss these options with them before proceeding. I also encourage you to do your own research on the topics as western medicine is not often inclusive of holistic or alternative approaches right away.

We are each in a different place and our needs are not identical to one another's, so what works for you might look a little different than what worked for me. As a detox, I drank my Blueberry Kale Smoothie 5 days a week for 6 weeks before expanding my breakfast horizons. It's still my favorite smoothie and if I feel the need to, I mix it with some granola and eat it with a spoon.

Avoid gluten and processed foods at lunch and opt for something like tuna with an avocado on lettuce or celery and nut butter. Snack on Trek Mix or Nuts, fruits and vegetables. A cucumber is so easy to grab, lob the ends off and eat. I love it as a snack on the go or even as part of breakfast. When I was starting out on this lifestyle, I was obsessed with the Broccoli Slaw and Kale Salad from Trader Joe's and ate it often. Any hearty salad with dark leafy greens would work just fine but avoid salads that are only iceberg and or romaine. We want dark leaves full of nutrients! Add a protein and you are set. As a general rule now, I do two vegetables, or a salad and a vegetable with protein for dinner. If I make grains, they are rice or quinoa.

It's a great idea, before you begin this new way of eating, to check in with how you feel currently. Here are some suggestions of what to record and monitor throughout this process. A visual reminder of progress is a great motivator! Measure and record each of these at the onset of your lifestyle change, then check in again after two weeks, then again after a month.

Weight
Blood Pressure
Body Fat Percentage
Quality of Sleep
Skin Clarity
Food Cravings
Regularity of Bowel Movements
Joint Pain
Energy Level

You have permission to eat like crazy, off of the list of anti-inflammatory foods. The idea is to get as many anti-inflammatory foods into you and as few inflammatory foods as possible. As this is not so much a diet as it is a lifestyle, I do not ask you to count calories or measure portions. Eating a ton of fresh pineapple everyday won't do you any good if it's on top of a pizza or next to your big bowl of cereal. Classify food choices based on whether they will add to your inflammation or take away from it. That said, if you are under the care of a doctor who is asking you to control your caloric intake, do it but with these foods.

Also, have fun experimenting with new food combinations! You'll be surprised at how easy it is to eat this way once you equip yourself to do it.

Remember: With everything you eat ask yourself if it will add inflammation to your body or take away inflammation.

Foods to Eat

A variety of foods have anti-inflammatory properties. Be sure to include plenty of them into your diet. These include foods that are high in antioxidants and polyphenols, such as:

- Vegetables: Broccoli, kale, Brussels sprouts, cabbage, cauliflower, etc.
- Fruit: Especially deeply colored berries like grapes and cherries.
- High-fat fruits: Avocados and olives.
- Healthy fats: Olive oil and coconut oil.
- Fatty fish: Salmon, sardines, herring, mackerel and anchovies.
- Nuts: Almonds, walnuts and other nuts.
- Peppers: Bell peppers and chili peppers.
- Chocolate: Dark chocolate.
- Spices: Such as turmeric, fenugreek and cinnamon.
- Tea: Green tea.

- Red wine: Up to 5 oz of red wine per day for women, and 10 oz per day for men.

What Not to Eat

- Sugary beverages: Sugar-sweetened drinks and fruit juices.
- Refined carbs: White bread, white pasta, etc.
- Desserts: Cookies, candy, cake and ice cream.
- Processed meat: Hot dogs, bologna, sausages, etc.
- Processed snack foods: Crackers, chips and pretzels.
- Certain oils: Processed seed- and vegetable oils like soybean and corn oil.
- Trans fats: Foods with "partially hydrogenated" in the ingredients list.
- Alcohol: Excessive alcohol consumption.
- Lard or Margarine
- Fried Foods

Anti-inflammatory Shopping List (4)

These foods are not the only fruits and vegetables that you can choose to eat. They just happen to be anti-inflammatory. By far, they should be your first choice foods. This diet is as much about what you add into it as it is what you take out, so you'll want to eat plenty of these beauties! As you select your food, ask yourself if it will add to your inflammation or take away the inflammation. Soon this will replace food choices based on craving. These lists are largely from Dr. William Davis's book, <u>Wheat Belly</u>.

Almond milk

Apples

Avocado

Berries- all, but blue are the best!

Broccoli

Beets

Bok Choy

Bone Broth

Celery

Chard

Cherries

Chia seeds

Coconut Milk

Coconut oil

Cauliflower

Dark Chocolate

Dried Fruit

Fatty Fish

Flaxseed—ground

Garlic
Ghee
Ginger
Grapes
Green Tea
Kale
Mackerel
Mushrooms
Nuts
Nut butters

Olive Oil
Oranges
Pineapple- Fresh!
Salmon
Shirataki noodles (in the refrigerated section)
Spinach
Tomato
Save all and any bones for bone broth!!!

Grain
Rice
Quinoa
Oats
Millet
Amaranth

Baking (4)

Almond meal, Almond Flour
Almond milk, unsweetened
Cocoa powder, unsweetened
Coconut flour
Coconut milk (canned and carton)
Coconut, shredded and unsweetened
Extracts—almond, coconut, vanilla
Ground nut meals—ground almonds, pecans, walnuts
—almond butter, peanut butter, sunflower seed butter

Nuts—raw almonds, pecans, walnuts, pistachios, hazelnuts, Brazil nuts; chopped walnuts or pecans for baking
Oils—extra-virgin olive, coconut, avocado, flaxseed, walnut
Sea salt
Sweeteners—liquid stevia, erythritol, Truvía, xylitol

Foods that contain wheat, which might surprise you

Baguettes	Graham Flour
Barley, barley wheat	Gravies
Beignets	Hydrolyzed Vegetable
Bran	protein
Brioche	Hydrolyzed wheat starch
Burritos	Kamut
Caramel coloring	Maltodextrin
Caramel flavoring	Matzo
Couscous	Modified food starch
Crepes	Orzo
Croutons	Panko
Dextrimaltose	Ramen
Dressings	Roux
Durum Wheat	Rusk
Einkorn	Rye
Emmer	Seasoning packets
Emulsifiers	Seitan
Farina	Semolina
Farro	Soba
Focaccia	Soy Sauce
Fu	Spelt
Gnocchi	Stabilizers

Tabbouleh

Tarts

Textured vegetable protein

Triticale

Triticum

Udon

Vital Wheat gluten

Wheat Bran

Wheat Germs

Wraps

Prebiotic Foods (36)(37)

Apples

Bananas

Chicory Root

Chickpeas

Cocoa

Dandelion Root

Flaxseed

Garlic

Grapefruit

Jerusalem Artichokes

Jicama Root

Leeks

Lentils

Oats

Onion

Red Kidney Beans

Savoy Cabbage

Seaweed

Shallots

Soybeans

Spring Onion

Watermelon

Probiotic Foods (38)(39)

Apple Cider Vinegar

Kiefer

Sauerkraut

Kimchi

Fermented Vegetables

Miso

Tempeh
Kombucha
Yogurt
Pickles

Assignment:

What are your initial thoughts after reading the anti-inflammatory foods list?

In which ways do you feel resistance to this way of eating?

Were there any emotions that arose within you? If so, what are they?

Is there a story behind those emotions?
What is it?

Whatever you wrote above, is exactly what you will need to pick apart and examine. Ask yourself how valid, and factual your statements are. Are they true? Could you have made a rule out of something that has occurred just once or twice? Examine your word choices. What do they tell you? We'll cover this in more detail on page

Assignment:

What are 5 meals you can think of right now off of those lists?
1.

2.

3.

4.

5.

What are 3 meals that you make for yourself now that you can easily modify to make anti-inflammatory?
1.

2.

3.

One way to add nutrition to a wide variety of your foods is to begin adding seeds to your diet. They can be added to just about anything and they really pack a punch nutritionally. Add them to your yogurt, smoothies, salads, steamed veggies, trek mixes, nutritional bars, avocado and just about anything else you think sounds like a good combination. The following section is a breakdown of different seeds and what they do for you.

Super Seeds!

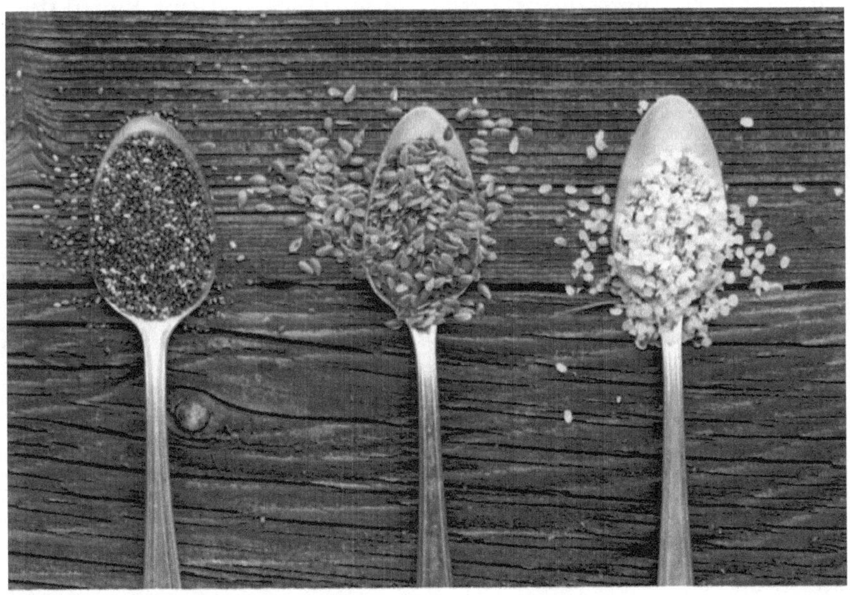

Alicia Cho/Thrive Market

Chia, flax and hemp seeds are all excellent additions to your diet. They blend well into smoothies (I love that nutty flax taste!), yogurts and granolas. They top salads, can be added to oatmeal or mixed in with your avocado spread. However you prefer them, these powerhouse seeds can significantly boost the nutrition of your meal.

Each of these seeds, however, pack different stores of nutrition. This is how they break down.

Hemp

Hemp seeds outshine chia and flax when it comes to protein: Two tablespoons serve up almost 7 grams, the amount found in two egg whites. Plus, the protein in hemp seeds contain all essential amino acids, which is unusual for plant foods. Hemp seeds are also an outstanding source of magnesium, a mineral that helps regulate blood pressure and blood sugar. Blend two tablespoons into your smoothie and you'll get one-quarter of a day's worth of magnesium (116 mg).

Chia

Chia seeds, also high in magnesium, have proven to be a good source of calcium; one serving offers 18% of your daily calcium intake. They also contain phosphorus, offering 27% of daily requirements. Where chia seeds really stand out however, is in the amount of fiber they contain, boasting 5 grams per tablespoon of whole seeds. These little beauties can absorb 10x their weight in water which is why Chia Seed Pudding can exist. Try it, you'll be in love.

Flax

While flax seeds need to be ground in order for you to reap their benefits, they contain something that the other two do not; lignans. Lignans are phytochemicals linked to breast and prostate cancer prevention. These seeds, the least expensive of the bunch, also contain the highest amount of omega-3 fatty acids.

	PROTEIN	CARBS	FAT	FIBER	FATTY ACIDS	AMINO ACIDS	VITAMINS	MINERALS
estimates based on 2 tbsp serving from self nutrition data								
CHIA	6 g	10 g	9 g	10 g	high in omega-3s	all essential amino acids	good source of thiamin (B1)	good source of calcium, magnesium and iron
FLAX	5 g	8 g	8 g	5 g	high in omega-3s	all essential amino acids	high in thiamin (B1)	high in magnesium, + good source of calcium, and iron
HEMP	6.8 g	<1 g	10 g	<1 g	1:1 ratio of omega-6 and omega-3	all amino acids	high in thiamin (B1) + good source of B6	high in magnesium, + good source of iron

Playing for Eats.com

Other Nutrition Packet Add In's
Goji Berries (Dried)

This antioxidant powerhouse not only protects your body against disease, but it also boosts brain health and is said to slow the aging process. Brimming with vitamin A the goji berry will support your immune system as well as your eye health. It's antioxidant effects help prevent heart disease. (12)

Pumpkin Seeds

Loaded with zinc, iron and protein, this fall favorite will fight to lower your cholesterol, strengthen your bones and immune system, as well as decrease the risk of certain types of cancer. (12)

Sesame Seeds

The plant compound sesamin has been shown to lower cholesterol, prevent high blood pressure, and protect the body from liver damage. According to Nutri-Bullet, just ¼ cup sesame seeds contains 35% of the daily recommended intake of calcium, and 73.5% of the daily recommended value of copper. (12)

Sunflower Seeds

These beauties are rich in phytosterol, a natural chemical that can lower your LDL cholesterol. They also contain vitamin E which helps prevent heart disease and relieves both arthritis and asthma, and selenium which repairs damaged cells, kills cancer cells and detoxifies the liver. (12)

A Bit About Food

Almond Flour/ Almond Meal-

The difference is that Almond Flour is made from ground blanched almonds while Almond Meal is made from ground whole almonds. Use Almond Flour for a lighter texture and Almond Meal, which is less expensive, for everyday use. (4)

Almond Milk, unsweetened-

You might also try hemp, soy, coconut or rice milk. Almond Milk is strained liquid from ground almonds and is a delicious milk substitute. (4)

Avocados

Packed with potassium, magnesium, fiber and heart-healthy monounsaturated fats, they also contain carotenoids and tocopherols, which are linked to reduced cancer risk. In addition, one compound in avocados may reduce inflammation in young skin cells. In one study, when people consumed a slice of avocado with a hamburger, they had lower levels of the inflammatory markers NF-kB and IL-6 than participants who ate the hamburger alone.

Berries

Berries contain antioxidants called anthocyanins. These compounds have anti-inflammatory effects that may reduce your risk of disease. Your body produces natural killer cells (NK cells), which help keep your immune system functioning properly. In one study, men who consumed blueberries every day produced significantly more NK cells than men who did not. In another study, overweight men and women who ate strawberries had lower levels of certain inflammatory markers associated with heart disease

Broccoli

Broccoli is extremely nutritious. It's a cruciferous vegetable, along with cauliflower, Brussels sprouts and kale.

Research has shown that eating a lot of cruciferous vegetables is associated with a decreased risk of heart disease and cancer. This may be related to the anti-inflammatory effects of the antioxidants they contain.

Broccoli is rich in sulforaphane, an antioxidant that fights inflammation by reducing your levels of cytokines and NF-kB, which drive inflammation.

Green, unripe Bananas

The unripe banana's sugars are in indigestible form and provide nutrition for bowel flora. (4)

Cauliflower

A great replacement for mashed potatoes and rice. Also makes a fantastic soup base! In fact, Cauliflower has become such a popular substitute for grains, you can find anything from cauliflower pizza dough to cauliflower crackers.

It is rich in vitamin C, potassium, vitamin B-6 and fiber. Full of antioxidants, including sulforaphane, and low in calories, this powerhouse veggie might become your new favorite.

Cherries

Cherries are delicious and rich in antioxidants, such as anthocyanins and catechins, which fight inflammation. Although the health-promoting properties of tart cherries have been studied more than other varieties, sweet cherries also provide benefits.

In one study, when people consumed 280 grams of cherries per day for one month, their levels of the inflammatory marker CRP decreased — and stayed low for 28 days after they stopped eating cherries.

Chia Seed

I love this seed! Use it to thicken smoothies, yogurts and kefirs. It also makes a fantastic pudding. No joke! I've even heard it used for mousses and jams.

Chocolate

Yes, chocolate! 100% chocolate- cocoa with cocoa butter and no sugar.

Coconut, Shredded and unsweetened; coconut flakes

Great for chewiness, texture and flavor in baking. An excellent addition to your morning custard.

Coconut Milk

A great replacement for cream and also an excellent thickening agent.

Cultures

Starting cultures for yogurts and kefirs can be purchased. I've heard making your own yogurt is easy and fun. I'll certainly be giving it a try.

Dark Chocolate and Cocoa

Dark chocolate is delicious, rich and satisfying. It's also packed with antioxidants that reduce inflammation. These may reduce your risk of disease and lead to healthier aging. Flavanols are responsible for chocolate's anti-inflammatory effects and keep the endothelial cells that line your arteries healthy. In one study, smokers experienced significant improvement in endothelial function two hours after eating high-flavanol chocolate. However, make sure to choose dark chocolate that contains at least 70% cocoa — more is even better — in order to reap the anti-inflammatory benefits.

Dried Fruit

Use them in baking, but make sure you buy the unsweetened kind!

Extra Virgin Olive Oil

Extra virgin olive oil is one of the healthiest fats you can eat. It's rich in monounsaturated fats and a staple in the Mediterranean diet, which provides numerous health benefits. Studies link extra virgin olive oil to a reduced risk of heart disease, brain cancer and other serious health conditions.

In one Mediterranean diet study, CRP and several other inflammatory markers significantly decreased in those who consumed 1.7 ounces (50 ml) of olive oil daily. The effect of oleocanthal, an antioxidant found in olive oil, has been compared to anti-inflammatory drugs like ibuprofen. Keep in mind that anti-inflammatory benefits are much greater in extra virgin olive oil than in more refined olive oils.

Extracts

Almond, Coconut, Vanilla, Lemon, Orange & Peppermint for baking.

Fatty Fish
Fatty fish are a great source of protein and the long-chain omega-3 fatty acids EPA and DHA. Although all types of fish contain some omega-3 fatty acids, these fatty fish are among the best sources:

- Salmon
- Sardines

- Herring
- Mackerel
- Anchovies

EPA and DHA reduce inflammation. Your body metabolizes these fatty acids into compounds called resolvins and protectins, which have anti-inflammatory effects. In clinical studies, people consuming salmon or EPA and DHA supplements had decreases in the inflammatory marker C-reactive protein (CRP). However, in another study, people with an irregular heartbeat who took EPA and DHA daily experienced no difference in inflammatory markers compared to those who received a placebo

Flaxseed

I love the flavor these add to my food! I've also added them to my water for a mild nutty flavor but mostly for the valuable Omega 3's. This is great mixed with almond flour for baking.

Ghee

AKA clarified butter. Most of the whey, casein, and lactose have been removed. Ghee is the oil from butter with the protein solids removed.

Grapes

Grapes contain anthocyanins, which reduce inflammation. In addition, they may decrease the risk of several diseases, including heart disease, diabetes, obesity, Alzheimer's disease and eye disorders. Grapes are also one of the best sources of resveratrol, another compound that has many health benefits. In one study, people with heart disease who consumed grape extract daily experienced a decrease in inflammatory gene markers, including NF-kB.

What's more, their levels of adiponectin increased. Low levels are associated with weight gain and an increased risk of cancer.

Green Tea

Green tea is one of the healthiest beverages you can drink. It reduces your risk of heart disease, cancer, Alzheimer's disease, obesity and other conditions. Many of its benefits are due to its antioxidant and anti-inflammatory properties, especially a substance called epigallocatechin-3-gallate (EGCG). EGCG inhibits inflammation by reducing pro-inflammatory cytokine production and damage to the fatty acids in your cells

Guar Gum

A thickener derived from the guar bean. It can be used with both hot and cold liquids.

Mushrooms

Mushrooms are very low in calories and rich in selenium, copper and all of the B vitamins. They also contain phenols and other antioxidants that provide anti-inflammatory protection. A special type of mushroom called lion's mane may potentially reduce the low-grade inflammation seen in obesity. As with most vegetables, cooking them lowers their anti-inflammatory compounds. These powerhouse fungi are best eaten raw or very lightly cooked.

Nut and Seed Butters

Rich in protein, healthy fats and fiber, nutty butters go well with almost anything! Put them in your smoothies, on your celery or apples or slather them on to a rice cake.

Nut meals and flours

Made with ground almonds, cashew, pecans, hazelnuts, walnuts these meals and flours are an excellent replacement for wheat flours.

Nuts

Always have them on hand! They are full of protein and fiber and will sustain you when your energy is low.

Oils

Extra virgin olive, coconut, flaxseed, walnut, and avocado oils are excellent choices.

Peppers

Bell peppers and chili peppers are loaded with vitamin C and antioxidants that have powerful anti-inflammatory effects. Bell peppers provide the antioxidant quercetin, which may reduce one marker of oxidative damage in people with sarcoidosis, an inflammatory disease. I love them with breakfast!

Chili peppers contain sinapic acid and ferulic acid, which may reduce inflammation and lead to healthier aging.

Seeds

Great for baking, granolas, salads and flours. Add them to your smoothie, your yogurt or your oatmeal. Seeds are packed with nutrition and easy to add into your menu.

Sweeteners

Pure liquid stevia, stevia glycerite, pure powdered stevia, powdered stevia with inulin, powdered erythritol, Swerve, Truvia, xylitol.

Tomatoes

The tomato is a nutritional powerhouse. Tomatoes are high in vitamin C, potassium and lycopene, an antioxidant with impressive anti-inflammatory properties. Lycopene may be particularly beneficial for reducing pro-inflammatory compounds related to several types of cancer. One study determined that drinking tomato juice significantly decreased inflammatory markers in overweight — but not obese — women. Note that cooking tomatoes in olive oil can maximize the amount of lycopene you absorb. That's because lycopene is a carotenoid, or a fat-soluble nutrient. Carotenoids are absorbed better with a source of fat.

Xanthan Gum

A fiber thickener which makes dough more cohesive and sturdier. Also used for making ice cream and iced coconut desserts.

Spice it up!

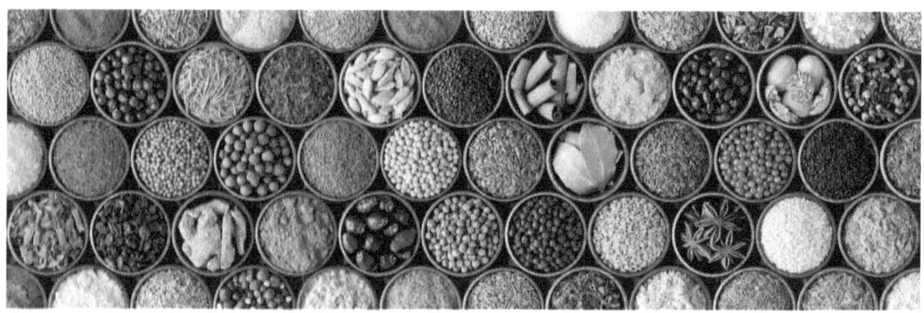

Turmeric

Turmeric is a spice with a strong, earthy flavor that's often used in curries and other Indian dishes. Lately, it has received a lot of attention for its content of the powerful anti-inflammatory nutrient curcumin.

Turmeric is effective at reducing the inflammation related to arthritis, diabetes and other diseases. One gram of curcumin daily combined with piperine from black pepper caused a significant decrease in the inflammatory marker CRP in people with metabolic syndrome. However, it may be hard to get enough curcumin to have a noticeable effect from turmeric alone. In one study, overweight women who took 2.8 grams of turmeric per day had no improvement in inflammatory markers. Taking supplements containing isolated curcumin is much more effective. Curcumin supplements are often combined with piperine, which can boost curcumin absorption by 2,000%.

Ginger

Ginger is a zesty spice used in many cuisines. You can buy it powdered or as a fresh root in most supermarkets. Ginger has been used as a traditional medicine to treat stomach upset, headaches, and infections. The anti-inflammatory properties of ginger have been praised for centuries, and scientific studies have confirmed it.

Cinnamon

Cinnamon, a popular spice often used to flavor baked treats and undisputedly delicious on buttered toast, is more than just a delicious additive in our cakes. Studies have shown that the spice has anti-inflammatory properties and can ease swelling. Keep a good supply of cinnamon on hand and sprinkle it in your coffee or tea, and on top of your breakfast cereal, into your morning custard, or on a baked apple.

Garlic

The anti-inflammatory properties of garlic have been proven to ease arthritis symptoms. A little bit can go a long way. Highly nutritious with very few calories, fresh garlic can be used in almost any savory dish for added flavor and health benefits. If the taste is too much for you, roast a head of garlic for a sweeter, milder flavor. For me garlic is like avocado; it goes with everything.

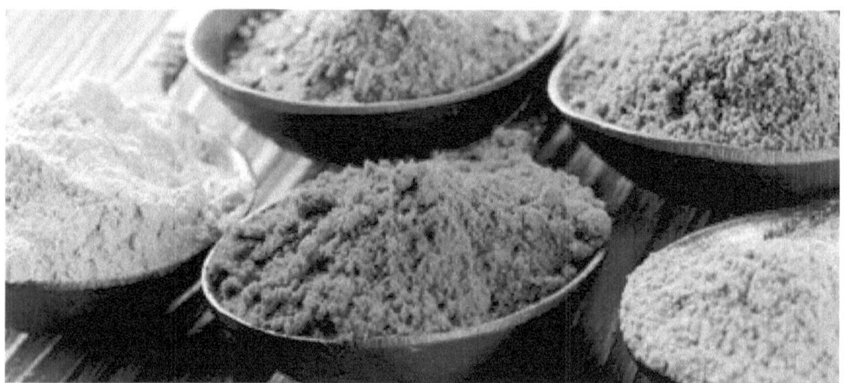

Cayenne

Cayenne and other hot chili peppers have been praised for their health benefits since ancient times. All chili peppers contain natural compounds called capsaicinoids. These are what give the spicy fruit its anti-inflammatory properties. Chili pepper is widely considered to be a powerful anti-inflammatory spice, so be sure to include a dash in your next dish. I love it in my bone broth. It has long been used as a digestive aid as well, so that's an added benefit.

Black pepper

If cayenne is too hot for your liking, you'll be happy to know that the milder black pepper has been identified for its anti-inflammatory properties as well. Known as the "King of Spices," black pepper has been valued for its flavor and antibacterial, antioxidant, and anti-inflammatory benefits. Studies have shown that the chemical compounds of black pepper, particularly piperine, may be effective in the early acute inflammatory process.

Clove (52)

Cloves have been used as an expectorant, and to treat upset stomach, nausea, and inflammation of the mouth and throat. Research is still mixed, but evidence suggests that they may have anti-inflammatory properties. Powdered clove works well in baked goods and in some savory dishes, like hearty soups and stews. You can also use whole cloves to infuse both flavor and nutrition into hot drinks like tea or cider.

Supplements

Boswellia

Lowers inflammation, fights joint pain, fights cancer, speeds up healing from infections, prevents autoimmune disease. (14)

Bromelain

May help prevent cancer, helps treat digestive disorders, supports faster recovery after surgery and injury, helps fight asthma and allergies, helps prevent and treat sinus infections, helps decrease joint pain, may aid in weight loss. (15)

Chondroitin

Glucosamine and chondroitin are structural components of cartilage, the tissue that cushions the joints. Both are produced naturally in the body. They are also available as dietary supplements. (16) Chondroitin is a major component in the fight against joint pain and osteoarthritis. It also helps in recovery after an injury.

Ginger

Ginger root contains gingerol its main component which is largely responsible for its anti-inflammatory and antioxidant powers. (17)

Ginger can greatly reduce the inflammatory response of osteoarthritis, calm a nauseous stomach (great for morning sickness), help with menstrual cramps, helps with muscles soreness, lowers blood sugars and reduces the risk for heart disease, can help with chronic indigestion, may improve brain function and reduce the risk for

Alzheimer's disease, may reduce the risk of cancer. ([17])

MSM (methylsulfonylmethane)

Is an organic sulfur containing compound that's used to improve immune function, lower inflammation and help restore healthy bodily tissue.

It is known to treat osteoarthritis and joint pain. It improves flexibility and restores collagen production in the joints. The MSM supplements help improve gut health and symptoms of leaky gut. It reduces skin problems such as rosacea and helps restore hair growth. MSM supplements are also known to reduce muscle soreness. ([18])

Omega-3

Getting enough Omega 3's are essential to optimal health. There are 3 types of fatty acids in your omega 3's; ALA, EPA, and DHA.

Omega 3's have been proven to fight depression, relieve anxiety, improve joint function and relieve the pain associated with osteoarthritis. Omega 3's are anti-inflammatory, improve brain health as well as eye health and will lower your risk for heart disease. Shown to improve mental health, Omega 3's also may prevent cancer and autoimmune disease. ([19])

Vitamin D

Known as the Sunshine Vitamin, vitamin D is produced by the body as a result of sun exposure ([20]). Vitamin D helps support healthy bones, immune system, nervous system. It reduces the risk of diabetes as well as the flu. ([20])

Probiotics

Probiotics are really one of the essential supplements to take as they add good flora into our guts. The cornerstone of our health is a healthy gut and probiotics are literally the soldiers in the trenches of our gut lining.

Proven to treat or prevent diarrhea, constipation, IBS, ulcerative colitis, Crohn's disease, H. pylori (the cause of ulcers), vaginal infections, urinary tract infections, recurrence of bladder cancer, infection of the digestive tract caused by Clostridium difficile, pouchitis (a possible side effect of surgery that removes the colon), eczema in children. (21)

Other effects of probiotics are that your immune system is boosted by them, you will probably lose weight as a side effect of the healthy gut they provide, and with more evidence mounting about our gut brain connection, some say taking probiotics help fight against depression and anxiety.

Prebiotics

Prebiotic fiber is a non-digestible part of foods like bananas, onions and garlic, Jerusalem artichoke, the skin of apples, chicory root, beans, and many others. Prebiotic fiber goes through the small intestine undigested and is fermented when it reaches the large colon. This fermentation process feeds beneficial bacteria colonies (including probiotic bacteria) and helps to increase the number of desirable bacteria in our digestive systems that are associated with better health and reduced disease risk.(22)

Collagen

Collagen, the most abundant protein in our bodies, is found in muscles, bones, skin, blood vessels, digestive system and tendons. (23)

Collagen improves health of skin and hair, reduces joint pains and degeneration, helps heal leaky gut, boosts metabolism, muscle mass and energy output, strengthens nails, hair and teeth, improves liver health, protects cardiovascular health. (23)

Hyaluronic Acid

Hyaluronic acid is a naturally occurring lubricant which is in high concentrations in the skin, joints, and eye fluids. A key function of hyaluronic acid is to help lubricate joints, skin, and the eyes. (24)

With the ability to absorb up to 1,000 times its weight in water, hyaluronic acid is a moisturizing mogul. It is known for promoting healthier, more supple skin. It fights off wrinkles too. It also, can speed wound healing, lubricate joints relieving joint pain, soothe acid reflux, relieve dry eyes and discomfort, preserving bone strength and combatting bladder pain and discomfort. (25)

They hydration factor alone makes this one of my favorite supplements, however, if you are nursing or battling cancer do not begin taking this supplement unless you have talked to your health care provider.

Glucosamine

Glucosamine produced in the body provides natural building blocks for growth, repair and maintenance of cartilage. Like chondroitin, glucosamine may lubricate joints, help cartilage retain water and prevent its breakdown. (26)

Glucosamine is used to treat a wide variety of inflammatory issues and is commonly known to fight joint and bone pain and inflammation. It is also used to help fight interstitial cystitis, inflammatory bowel disease, multiple sclerosis, glaucoma, temporomandibular joint (TMJ). (27)

Gelatin

Gelatin is what collagen breaks down into. Bone broth is known as an excellent way to consume collagen. You'll notice that a good bone broth will become gelatinous once put in the refrigerator overnight. That's because the collagen has been seeped from the bones and joints and in the process, it has been broken down into gelatin. This is not the sugar-filled flavored gelatin many of us love, rather it is a pure form of broken-down collagen. We are not beholden to only buy flavored, sugar-filled gelatin; pure gelatin is available and there are many fun ways to include it into your diet.

Turmeric

Despite its use in cooking for several thousand years, turmeric continues to surprise researchers in terms of its wide-ranging health benefits. While once focused on anti-inflammatory benefits, decreased cancer risk, and support of detoxification, studies on turmeric intake now include its potential for improving cognitive function, blood sugar balance, and kidney function, as well as lessening the degree of severity associated with certain forms of arthritis and certain digestive disorders. (28)

Fiber

Fiber should be a major part of our diet, sourced from whole plant foods. It not only feeds the good bacteria in our gut, improving gut health, but it also acts like a scrub brush in our system, pushing impurities out of our bodies. It will help maintain regular, healthy bowel movements, lower your cholesterol levels and even out your blood sugar levels. (29)

Slippery Elm

Slippery elm contains mucilage, a substance that becomes a slick gel when mixed with water. According to Dr. Axe, this mucilage coats and soothes the mouth, throat, stomach and intestines, making it ideal for sore throat, cough, gastroesophageal reflux disease (GERD), Crohn's disease, ulcerative colitis, irritable bowel syndrome (IBS), diverticulitis and diarrhea. Plus, it's been used to treat breast cancer! (30)

Over-the-Counter Medications

Over-the-counter (OTC) medications are drugs you can buy without a doctor's prescription. Nonsteroidal anti-inflammatory drugs (NSAIDs) are drugs that help reduce inflammation, which often helps to relieve pain. They are commonly used to fight inflammation.

Some of the more common NSAIDs are:
- aspirin
- ibuprofen (Advil, Motrin, Midol)
- naproxen (Aleve, Naprosyn)

NSAIDs can be very effective. They tend to work quickly and generally have fewer side effects than corticosteroids, which also help with inflammation. However, before you use an NSAID, you should know about the potential side effects and how they interact with other drugs.

NSAIDs block prostaglandins, a substance that sensitizes your nerve endings and enhances pain during inflammation. Prostaglandins also play a role in controlling your body temperature. By blocking these effects, NSAIDs help relieve your pain and bring down your fever.

In fact, NSAIDs can be helpful in reducing many types of discomfort, including:
- headache
- backache
- muscle aches
- inflammation and stiffness caused by arthritis and other inflammatory conditions

- menstrual aches and pains
- pain after a minor surgery
- sprains or other injuries

If you're at risk of heart attack or stroke, your doctor may recommend daily low-dose aspirin to help lower your risk.

Just because you can buy NSAIDs without a prescription doesn't mean they're perfectly safe. There are some potential side effects and risks.

Some of the most commonly reported side effects include stomach upset, diarrhea, and gas. You can minimize these side effects by taking your medication with food, milk, or antacids. Less often, NSAIDs may cause lightheadedness, dizziness, or mild headache.

Serious side effects that require immediate medical attention include:

- ringing in your ears
- blurry vision
- rash, hives, and itching
- fluid retention
- blood in your urine or stools
- vomiting and blood in your vomit
- severe stomach pain
- chest pain
- rapid heartbeat
- jaundice (yellowing of the skin and eyes)

NSAIDs are intended for occasional and short-term use. Your risk of side effects increases the longer you use them. So often when people have chronic inflammation, they resort to taking NSAIDs daily. While temporary pain relief is offered, damage to the stomach and intestinal lining that occurs actually creates more inflammation.

Children younger than 18 years who may have chickenpox or influenza should avoid aspirin and products containing aspirin. Giving aspirin to children can increase their risk of Reye's syndrome, which may result in liver and brain damage. Reye's syndrome is potentially fatal.

Some OTC medications, like acetaminophen (Tylenol) are good for relieving pain, but they don't help with inflammation.

You should also talk to your doctor about the safety of using an NSAID if you consume three or more alcoholic beverages a day or if you take blood thinning medications

The Benefits of Bone Broth

Collagen

Bone broth is the best source of natural collagen available to us. When the bones are boiled, all of the gelatin (which breaks down into cartilage) seeps out of the bone, it's marrow, joints and tendons and into the broth. A really good bone broth will gelatinize overnight.

Nutrient dense, this ancient and delicious comfort food will boost your immunity and add collagen (which begins to deplete after 40) to your body.

As a rich source of collagen, bone broth is good for your joints, hair, skin and nails.

Gut repair

That's right, the same gelatin that was seeped from the bones is responsible for strengthening and tightening gut lining. It fights food sensitivities and helps with the growth of beneficial probiotics. The collagen, which the gelatin breaks down into, provides amino acids, particularly glutamine, which support inflammation relief in the intestines.

Joint protection

The collagen in bone broth is extremely important to our joint health. As we age, we lose cartilage due to stress and shrinking. The collagen strengthens the cartilage and protects it from stress. Collagen may also help with the pain, stiffness and reduced range of motion associated with Osteoarthritis.

Improves sleep

Another amino acid provided by gelatin is, glycine. Bone broth is rich in this beautiful, anti-inflammatory amino acid that helps promote a good night's sleep as well as fight off daytime fatigue.

Supports weight loss

Sipping on bone broth before dinner each night will naturally reduce the amount of calories you intake. Also, bone broth is anti-inflammatory and as you lose inflammation, you will also lose weight.

Celery Juice

Consuming 16 ounces of pure, fresh celery juice each morning has grown in popularity as a powerful method of healing. It has been highly effective as celery is a powerful antioxidant which removes free radicals in the body. Consuming antioxidant foods can potentially decrease the risks of getting cancer. Additionally, celery can prevent cardiovascular diseases, jaundice, liver disease, urinary tract obstruction, gout, and rheumatic disorders. Celery can even reduce blood sugar levels, blood lipids, and blood pressure. Experimental studies show that celery has antifungal, antibacterial, and anti-inflammatory properties. Celery seeds have even been used in the treatment of skin conditions including psoriasis, and respiratory diseases including asthma and bronchitis.

Anthony Williams, The Medical Medium, is famous for advocating the amazing healing properties of celery juice. His knowledge of the healing power of food is remarkable and I recommend his books.

It must be said however, that while juicing is a highly efficient way to pack your body with nutrients, it can lead to some problems if you are not also taking care of the rest of your nutrition. When you juice, you are stripping the vegetable of its natural fiber; fiber which is an important part of your digestive process. You must be sure that you are getting adequate fiber from another source if you are going to be juicing regularly. Crunchy veggies, fruit, nuts and berries are all fibrous. With this lifestyle, you have plenty of opportunity to intake fiber.

Meal Plans

It's easier to stick to a diet when you have a plan. Here's a great sample menu to start from, featuring a day of anti-inflammatory meals:

1
Breakfast
Blueberry Kale Smoothie

Snack
Mixed Nuts

Lunch
Mixed green lettuce
Tuna mixed with turmeric, pepper, and sliced almonds
Celery with nut butter

Dinner
Grilled chicken w lemon
Sautéed spinach with garlic
Brussel sprouts
Quinoa

2

Breakfast
3 egg omelet with 1 cup mushrooms and
1 cup kale, cooked in coconut oil.
1 cup cherries.
Green tea, coffee and/or water.

Lunch
Grilled salmon on a bed of mixed greens
with olive oil and vinegar.
1 cup raspberries topped with plain Greek
yogurt and chopped pecans.
Iced tea, water.

Snack
Bell pepper strips with guacamole.

Dinner
Chicken curry with sweet potatoes, cauliflower and broccoli.
Red wine (5–10 oz or 140–280 g).
Dark chocolate (preferably at least 80% cocoa).

3

Breakfast
Coffee
Oatmeal with almond milk and topped with
blueberries, ground flaxseeds, and cinnamon
A banana

Snack
Almonds or Trek Mix
Celery

Lunch
Spinach salad with cherry tomatoes and tuna, with an extra-virgin olive oil and lemon juice dressing ...other things to add..hardboiled egg, celery, onion, almond slices.

Afternoon Snack
Green tea with fresh ginger or Kombucha or Mineral Water
An avocado cracked black pepper and red chili flakes...or whatever else you like on your avi.

Dinner
Stir Fry- Steak or Chicken w Snap Peas, Red Bell Pepper, Onion, Garlic, Ginger, Bean Sprouts over Quinoa or rice- No Soy Sauce!!!

Lifestyle

Lifestyle choices also contribute to the onset of chronic inflammation. A regular routine of working out will push toxins out of your body as you perspire. Beyond conditioning your heart and cardiovascular system, more than pushing unwanted toxins out of your body, regular exercise will help you to destress, regulate your hormones and kick your endorphin levels up a notch which will make you a happier person.

Obesity leads to chronic inflammation as does a lifestyle of stress. Exercise helps with both. We were made to move! While I know all too well how nice it is to stay cozy and not workout, the malaise is just a thin layer, like a crust, that you just have to break through. Once, you've gotten up and have busted through that layer, your body, mind and spirit will become reinvigorated and thankful to you.

Another major contributor to inflammation is stress. Anxiety, fear of the unknown, pressures from work and from relationships all add up and take an emotion and physical toll on our bodies. We were not meant to live a lifestyle of stress! We were not meant to sit in front of a screen or in traffic for the amount of time many of us do.

We were built to move. We were made for the sunshine and soil. This is not to say that we do not need economy, and we do not need to work. For many however, there is a lack of balance between the amount of stress that consumes us, lack of movement, and spending time outdoors, moving our bodies and de-stressing.

Going outdoors, even if it's just for a moment, can transform your day. Moving, sweating, breathing outdoors can transform your life. Not only have the benefits of being in nature been well documented, but it's logical from the standpoint that we are natural beings ourselves. False light, concrete and computer screens detach us, drain our energy, can lead to depression as well as anxiety, whereas being outdoors and making contact with nature has proven benefits in every area of life, including reduction of anxiety and stress.

Meditation

Where you focus and what you say about yourself matter quite a bit. Quieting your mind, praying, meditating and visualizing are all extremely valuable and important practices and can help you tune into your mindset and into what you are believing about yourself.

In each and every bit of the emotional spectrum, far and wide, your mind and your body are speaking to one another. A healthy gut biome will allow for a more clear, focused mind, as will the regular practice of meditation. With the practice of prayer and/or meditation you will notice as you quiet your mind and stop the ceaseless talking in your head, the spinning on issues, that you become less anxious, your body feels more relaxed and that you are in tune with what is going on in you and around you.

I wonder what your faith has to say about it.
Your intuition.

Your journey is yours and I respect it. I do want you to know that meditation has proven physical benefits.

Including:(41)(42)(43)

Reduced stress
Reduced anxiety
Reduced disorders related to anxiety
Reduced depression

Reduced inflammation
Enhanced self-awareness
Improved focus
Improved sleep
Helps control pain
Improved blood pressure
Increased empathy
Increased immunity
Boosts happiness
Improves memory

Meditation does not need to be a spiritual practice so much as a necessary quieting of your mind. There are many apps and videos that teach and guide meditations. If you are new to meditation, these are a great way to begin. I'm also available to help. The benefits of meditation are well documented, and it is something you can do today to improve your wellbeing.

Although it does not have to be a practice of spirituality, meditation lends itself perfectly to a spiritual life regardless of your faith.

One simple way to meditate is to sit quietly with good posture, clear your mind, and focus on your breathing. As you do this, focus on the breath drawing up from deep in your core, filling your lungs, rising into your chest and up into your head before you release the air back into the environment. Continue to focus on your life-giving breath as it energizes your body. If your mind wanders, it's okay, just let the thought be released and focus once again on your breathing.

For some, focusing on a scripture verse, a blessing or mantra that you repeat slowly as you breath is a form of meditation. You might repeat, "Abba" on my inhale and "Father" on the exhale. For others picturing a ball bearing, or a flame, a beach or really, anything that works, while focusing on breathing and turning off the constant stream of chattering is what brings them into meditation.

There are many ways to meditate and all of them bring the health and mental benefits described above. I encourage you to set aside 10 minutes each day towards this discipline. When you first start, it may be difficult to meditate for even 2 minutes, but as you practice you will find that 10 minutes will go quickly, and you will want to increase the amount of time you spend meditating.

Visualization

A natural mate for meditation is visualization. Top athletes and CEOs alike use this tool as a means to accomplish specific goals. (54) The idea is to visualize the ideal outcome and the actions that lead to it in as much detail as possible. Engage your senses as you do this. What is the weather like? Can you feel the sun on your back? The breeze in the air? What does the air smell like? Is there sweat on your brow? What noise is in the background? What emotion fills you in this ideal moment? What is your state of mind?

Across the board, successful people, top performers and those who have seen miraculous changes in their health openly embrace visualization as a means to better their outcomes. It is effective. Multiple studies have shown that our brains do not differentiate between an actual memory and a made up one. (57) When we visualize an action, the same regions of our brains light up as when we actually perform the action, thus neural networks are created. (58) The more time you can spend visualizing in vivid detail, your desired result, the stronger your connections become and the better your actual performance will be. I give you permission to express awe and wonder here, at our brains, they are fascinating! Life is fascinating!

In terms of health, go into as much detail as possible about what you would like to achieve. For some this might mean an actual vision of your cells becoming clean. Perhaps you can picture the inflammation leaving your body. Can you feel it? What does it feel like? What are your emotions surrounding this change? Is there a difference in how your body works? Connect emotionally with your desired outcome.

This is what you do:

1. Close your eyes and mentally set your intention on your goal.
2. State your goal in a positive and affirming way.
3. In as much detail as possible visualize your desired outcome. Use all five senses to create the vision.
4. Connect emotionally with your desired result. How does it feel? What are your emotions around it?

5.   Repeat frequently.

Creating a healthy and balanced life is a matter of spirit, mind and body. Releasing anxiety of the unknown and fear is one way to reduce stress and inflammation. Coupled with your faith, meditation and visualization are excellent practices within an anti-inflammatory lifestyle.

Assignment:

With this question please keep in mind that I'm asking you to be as real as possible. "Ideal" does not mean if you could suddenly transform your body into what society deems ideal, would you and what would that be. I do mean "ideal" for you. That might mean having legs that function correctly or sinuses that are no longer congested.

Please answer in as much detail as possible.
In terms of your body:

What does ideal look like?

What does ideal feel like?

What emotions come to the surface when you connect emotionally to your ideal?

Daily, I want you to connect emotionally with what you are heading towards. See yourself functioning the way you want to. Connect emotionally and energetically with the ideal version of yourself. Choose words that encourage and motivate you and feel great knowing that you are taking charge of your health!

Words!!

From forging nations to agreements among friends, to business transactions, words literally shape our world. Our relationship to them however, is more intimate, more powerful and more life shaping than many of us realize.

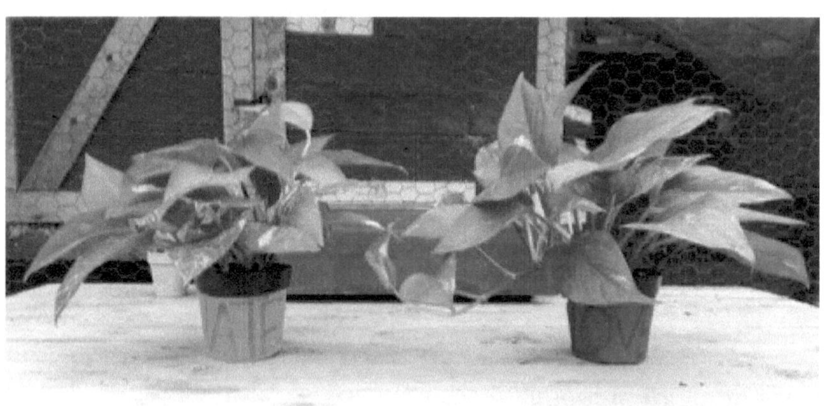

Fascinated by Dr. Emotos study on water, I decided to run a similar study that I had heard also demonstrates the power of our words. For about 6 months now I've been loving on one of these plants: speaking to it kindly telling it how beautiful it is and how well it is thriving. I bless the plant. The purpose of the second plant is to live a sad life where it is told it is no good and it's weak. I yell at this plant and swear at. To be honest though, I don't think there is enough hate in my house to truly stunt the "Hate" plant. Often days would go by without a word to the plants from me, let alone intention. I wrote "Love" and "Hate" on them as the written word also carries the energy of the intent behind it. Like all words, the words we speak over ourselves are tremendously powerful!

Have you read Dr. Emotos study on water yet (<u>59</u>)? If you haven't, please do so now! Really, it's fascinating. If the energy behind our words shapes the molecules in the water, imagine what they do to our bodies! We are 60% water on average. That's over half of our being that is being shaped by the energy and intent pointed towards it in the form of words. Imagine what it does to our food when we bless it, treat it well and with dignity. Is it any wonder so many of us are taught to bless our food before we eat!

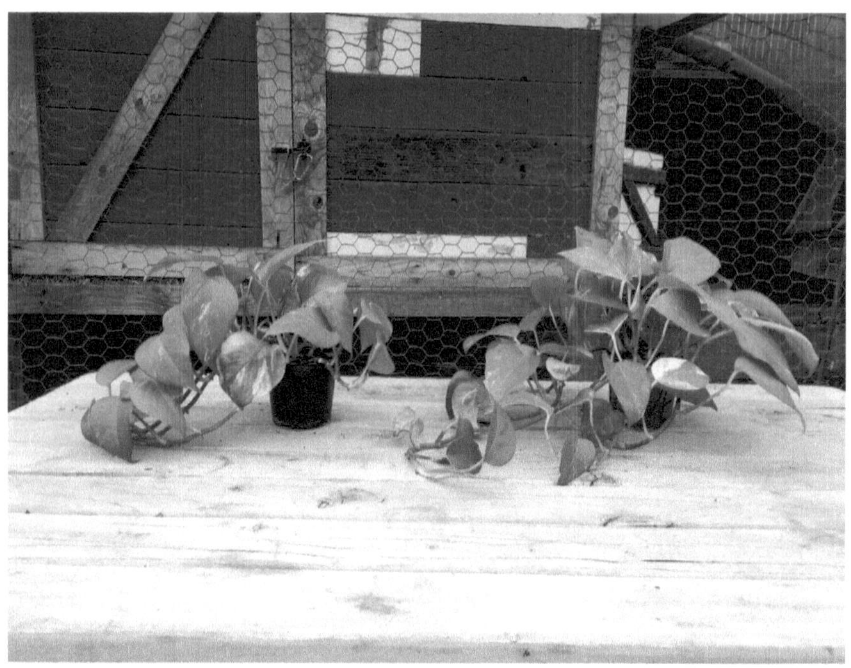

The world's religions have much to say about our words and our tongue and holding our thoughts captive. I'm still studying some and gathering information, but from a Judeau Christian perspective, God "spoke the world into being". If you consider that according to the same perspective we are also made in God's image, words take on a whole lot of power. Similarly, in Hinduism the world begins with a sound: OM.

In the same light, the Buddhist text The Dhammapada begins like this:

"What we are today comes from our thoughts of yesterday, and our present thoughts build our life of tomorrow: our life is the creation of our mind.

If a man speaks or acts with an impure mind, suffering follows him as the wheel of the cart follows the beast that draws the cart.

"What we are today comes from our thoughts of yesterday, and our present thoughts build our life of tomorrow: our life is a creation of our mind.

If a man speaks or acts with a pure mind, joy follows him as his own shadow."

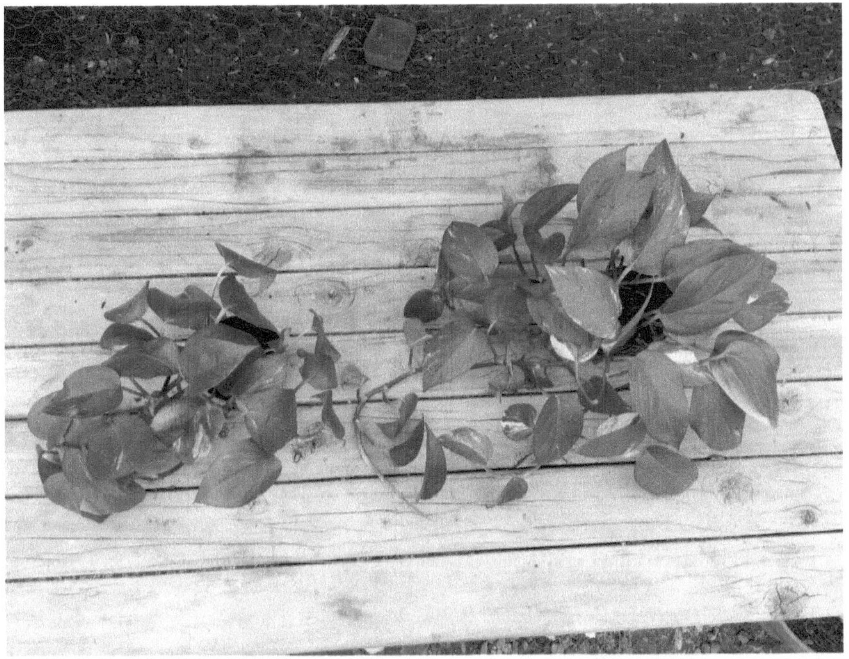

These plants are a beautiful demonstration of how words can stunt or encourage growth, and we'll keep watching them grow. In today's society we absolutely must connect and love and be kind to the people around us. There are so many people who can't connect due to their wounds compiled with their own words of self loathing that are repeated, thus anchored into their subconscious. From these wounded places they are deeply unhappy and may hurt people around them. We must bring connection and love into our communities! It begins with how we treat and love ourselves. We must become like the taproot, digging deep, gathering nourishment and supporting the rest of the root system.

Mindset

Rather than looking at going anti-inflammatory as a list of what you can't eat, open yourself up to all that you CAN eat. In fact, the more anti-inflammatory foods you can get into your body, the better off you will be. There is no calorie counting involved here. Just a whole lot of protein and greens, with a good measure of healthy fats.

I have known for a long time that diets and I are NOT compatible. I do not do well when being asked to measure my food or eat certain foods at certain times. My instant reaction is to push back whenever I feel restricted in anyway, so pah-leese do not tell me what to eat. I know many of you are the same way.

Going anti-inflammatory has worked for me, however, because I view this as eating for my health, not as a strict diet. I feel so great when I'm on it that I haven't even once in the near decade I've eaten this way, chosen to eat a bowl of pasta over alleviating my pain. I believe it is, in part, this subtle shift in mindset that allows for my success. We literally are what we eat. Your body will react to a change in what you put in it. The more you can focus on the multitude of results you will feel and the freedom to eat as much as you want whenever you want, the more excellent your results will be.

Intuitive Eating

We were all born with the knowledge of how to eat. Many fad diets over the years have stressed portion control, measuring your food and counting calories. For most, the idea of dieting means being told what to eat and in what quantity, this is the complete opposite of intuitive eating. Intuitive eating means listening to your body and what it's telling you about what your nutritional needs are.

When you break the cycle of craving wheat and sugar products and you begin to tune into your body, it becomes easy to decipher what it is telling you. The Original Intuitive Eating Pros have established the 10 Principles of Intuitive Eating. (60) They are

1. Reject the Diet Mentality
2. Honor your Hunger
3. Make Peace with Food
4. Challenge the Food Police
5. Respect your fullness
6. Discover the satisfaction Factor
7. Honor your feelings without using Food
8. Respect your Body
9. Exercise- Feel the Difference
10. Honor your Health

In marveling at how amazing our world is, it must be acknowledged that of course our bodies are fine-tuned, complex and so entirely off the hook amazing enough to know how they need to be nourished. It need not be said that once you are eating natural, anti-inflammatory foods and have eliminated cravings for foods that cause inflammation, your body will clearly tell you what foods it needs. It is these naturally sourced foods that your body will be calling for. You will know when you need protein, or greens, or fruit. You will know when you are satisfied and will not be overeating. Connect emotionally on this idea for a moment. Take some time here to be grateful for the beauty of our connection with all things natural. Wonder at it.

Preparing for Success

Have you ever confused self-care for self-indulgence? The two are easy to mix up.

This confusion shows up in the form of avoidance or self-numbing and it is truly not self-care. I think we've all be guilty of choosing to do something that feels good in the moment, but in the long run it is destructive.

You might think buying yourself something nice is going to make you feel better, but your empty pocketbook is saying something different.

Or perhaps you indulge in a vice, whether it's food, drugs, binge watching on Amazon, or staring at your phone for 2 hours thinking you deserve it, when really it makes you feel guilty, unempowered and sluggish.

You reach for that second doughnut (or first!) and enjoy the sugar fix but feel guilty about it later. Is that self-care?

True self-care would have been choosing to not spend money that you don't have or choosing to workout rather than indulge. True self care is doing something that you might have resistance toward at first, but which makes you feel great after.

They key here is tapping into how the behavior, habit, indulgence makes you feel after it's done. Do you feel refreshed or guilty? Did it add to your self-confidence or make you a little ashamed?

Listen to your emotions. Listen to your body.

True self care is doing the things that are healthy and refreshing to your spirit, mind and body.

You will know you are doing these because of how you feel afterwards.

I've never once regretted a walk on the beach, a hike, a workout, cranking the tunes and dancing, practicing a craft, helping a neighbor, stretching out on the floor, or cleaning my home.

Assignment:

What is one thing you do under the guise of self-care, that is truly avoidance, numbing yourself or indulgence.

What is 1 activity that you never regret?

Choosing to love yourself means actual self-care. Choose to do those things that fill you. Make the choice to participate in activities that feel good after the fact, not just in the moment.

List 3 activities you can choose to do which you never regret
1.
2.
3.

Assignment:

Have you successfully made major dietary changes before?

What has worked for you in the past?

What is motivating you now?

For some, this change will be an easy transition; fine tuning on a journey that you're familiar with.

For others, however, this might be another attempt in a series of many to gain control of your nutrition; a battle you've begun and abandoned many times.

Inflammation is everywhere, in your sore hip, cracking knees, digestive issues, skin issues and major disease alike. Maybe you are just like so many who know that a dietary change will make a big difference in how you feel daily. We want to age well and be able to enjoy our lives. You know it's important to be proactive and you're ready to begin.

For many, there is a version of you that you dream about living out, but your reality looks nothing like it. You are strong, capable and ready to capture the world by storm on the inside, but are buried in extra weight that you know doesn't belong on your amazing self, your body is beginning to hurt and you are continuing to put yourself down for it.

Regardless of what your story is, once you decide to make this change you must accept that it is a journey, ongoing. You must be gentle and kind to yourself and to your body because none of us are perfect all the time. Holding onto anger at yourself and others, is toxic to your spirit, mind and body. This is truly a decision to love yourself and to do so properly is to be kind, forgiving and...well, loving to your whole being.

What Drives Us

Knowing what you need to do is only a part of your journey to wellness. It's actually doing what you need to do with consistency that will determine your outcomes. This sounds so obvious and it is rather simple, but why then does it so often turn into such a challenge?

You know that dairy upsets your stomach, but you eat the ice cream anyway.

Moments before releasing the yogurt cup into the trash you realize it actually belongs in recycling, yet you follow through with your momentum and drop it in the trash anyway. Of course, you then have to fish it out of the trash can and put it in recycling.

You know sitting on the couch after sitting all day at work contributes to your back pain, and that a walk would be better for you, yet you find yourself on the couch, remote in hand night after night.

You reach for the second doughnut even though you know sugar is the enemy.

If you are really ready to make a change, you'll need to identify the barriers which are standing in your way. What makes you do one thing, when you know you should do another?

This is what is going on: We might KNOW on a conscious level what the healthy decision is, but we ACT based on what our subconscious believes.

When you were a baby, your subconscious was wide open to the beliefs that your family and surrounding environment put into it. If you grew up in scarcity you might have a deeply held belief that there won't be enough food or enough money. If you were rewarded with food, you might associate it with praise from your mom or dad.

You did not choose the beliefs your subconscious has gathered but your mind is holding onto them tightly and is driving your actions based on those beliefs. In fact, your subconscious would do just about anything to protect you and theses beliefs. They are the framework of your reality.

The key to figuring out your deeply held, subconscious beliefs lies within your words, the stories you believe about yourself, and the emotions that are connected to them.

Assignment:

Was your Mom or Dad obsessed with being thin? Fat? Sick? Healthy?

What were the predominant attitudes that you grew up with surround food, health, living holistically?

Our subconscious is a tricky thing, but not so dubious it can't be rewired. Going into this, pay attention to your mindset and to any emotions that arise surrounding the lifestyle change. Listen to how you describe your health journey, your body, fitness level, sleep patterns, food choices as this is where your subconscious beliefs hide. Listen carefully to the words you use about yourself and the stories you use to justify them. What you repeat over and over again about yourself has been written, through repetition into your subconscious as well.

You may need to rearrange some thought patterns, eliminate negative ones and create new, empowering ones. These changes may be a drastic shift from, "I hate my body", to "I love that my body is getting stronger every day." Or maybe it's, "This disease is bringing me down", to "I eat so clean that, this disease is going down!". According to Jen Sincero, our words bring our thoughts and beliefs to life. Our thoughts become our words, our words become our beliefs, our beliefs become our actions, our actions become our habits and our habits become our realities. (31)

Our words are so very powerful! How we speak about our bodies, our nutrition, or success, plays a tremendous role in our ultimate outcome. The picture that we paint of ourselves so often dictates how we actually are. Owning your positive new way of eating, connecting emotionally with your success, and tapping into what your body and mind are telling you will set you up for success.

Too often we go throughout our day caught in our heads. Events happen which fill us with everything from elation to rage. Often it is hard to let go of events and the emotions that go with them. We think about things that have happened in the past, which we have no control of, rather than pointing our energy to the future and being present in the moment. We talk to ourselves about everything, non-stop. We have the ability to replay moments, over and over and over again. We debate issues with ourselves. We go over the things we "need to do", or "should have" done differently. We criticize ourselves and others too at times.

Assignment:

Have you ever held onto an issue surrounding your health and replayed it over and over again?

What emotions were arising at that time?

What emotions arise now?

What got you through it?

Focus

The direction we choose to focus our thoughts literally creates our reality. Our thoughts turn into our words and our words turn into action. Wherever you place your focus is going to be where you see development in your life.

It is so simple and yet so difficult, especially when your head won't quiet down and you keep replaying that emotional conversation with the ex, which happened 3 weeks ago (but you can't seem to let it go), or your worried about how to pay the bills, or your nagging stomach cramps are back again. Particularly if you are in the habit of saying negative things about your body, ranging from mildly negative to extremely negative and self-deprecating. We are all in different places in life and if you want to change where you are right now, regarding your body and health issues, you can. The key to your success begins in your mind.

Reframing how we speak to ourselves and the stories that we believe about ourselves is extremely powerful. Our words are extremely powerful! When we repeat something to ourselves over and over again, we anchor in the belief that it's true and we draw more of it to ourselves. If you are going to gain control of your health and wellness, you need to be clear on what you are believing about yourself. You'll need to be objective and analyze whether the statement is actually true or not. Pick it apart, take away its powers.

Example:

"I hate my stomach. It'll always be huge."

Is that true? Do you honestly hate the part of you which is literally the core of your body? It's the part that receives food! Is "HATE" the right word? Is it the size that you don't like?

Really? It'll "ALWAYS be huge"? Well, I guess that depends on which actions you take and don't take. Has no one ever lost their huge stomachs? Are there not a gillion examples on Instagram about body transformations? We know the right nutrition. Have you done all the right things with consistency?

When you catch yourself beginning the negative statement, STOP, call it out as untrue, and replace it with something better.

The example above could be:

"I'm in control of this. I know what to do and I'm kicking ass doing it!" Or, "I love my stomach and I'm going to show my love by taking care of it from the inside out."

This is a great time to connect emotionally to your final outcome.

Here is another example:

"Everyone in my family has arthritis. I'm doomed!"

This can become:

"There is a lot of arthritis in my family, but I'm eating so clean now, and being so proactive. I feel like I'm really going to win this through good nutrition."

Assignment:

Take a week and listen to how you speak to yourself. What negative statement or name have you used regarding yourself? Your life? Your age? Your body?

What are 3 things that you say to yourself that you would like to change?

Where did those statements and thoughts come from?

What will you change them to?

As you move into this new way of eating, check in with yourself periodically to notice changes in how your body feels. Within a few to several weeks or months (it's different for everybody), you will soon find yourself focusing on how good you feel.

Louise Hay is famous for her affirmations. She is well respected and has a lot of wisdom to share. This is an exercise she introduced me to through her book, <u>You Can Heal Your Life.</u>

Right now, I challenge you to look deeply into your own eyes, in front of a mirror. Can you maintain steady eye contact with yourself? I challenge you to say this to yourself out loud.

"I love you. I deserve this change. I can do this. I WILL do this!

I love you, I love you, I love you, I love you, I love you, I love you, I love you, I love you, I love you, I love you!" (that's 10 times...).

This is a simple task, but it's not always easy. Often, emotions arise while one speaks to themselves in the mirror. This can be a powerful tool for getting to the root of subconscious beliefs.

Assignment:

If this was an emotional experience, take a moment to write down how you feel and why.

Is what you have to say true from an objective standpoint?

What is the root of these beliefs?

What phrases, questions or words do you find yourself using around this issue?

When you find yourself using these negative words or phrases, call them out immediately as lies. After you've called them out replace them with empowering words. Let these words become your new truths.

Often our body, weight, health issues are seated deeply in our subconscious mind. Often when we do tune into the stories we believe about ourselves, emotions also come to the surface. Often painful memories that need to be examined, picked apart and discarded are tied to these beliefs about ourselves. It's time to dig deep, unbury the junk and own your story and your health. You do deserve to be healthy. You do deserve this change and you CAN do it.

I also want you to stand with the confidence and strength you will feel once you begin to shape your life into what you want it to be. Stand in this position in front of the mirror. Connect emotionally. Carry yourself through the day as if you already have what you are after.

Assignment:

Think about your current health situation that you would like to see change. Write in as much detail as you possible, situation you deal with regularly surrounding your health. For instance, maybe it's become increasingly difficult and painful to go up a flight of stairs. Or perhaps your arthritis is making it difficult and painful to use your hands effectively. Maybe you feel badly about yourself, calling yourself old and weak each day as you watch young students play basketball. Write about what goes on as well as what you feel and how you feel in the moment. Write all about the situation as it is.

On a separate sheet of paper write about the same situation but this time write it as you would like it to be. Write in as much detail as possible what goes on as well as what you feel and how you feel in the moment.

Burn the first one.

It's extremely important to connect emotionally with the second version of your story. Each day feel the success you've had with the diet, even if it's your very first day. Truly connect on an emotional level with the success you will see with this new way of eating. Be proud that you are feeding your body natural foods, grown from the earth, not in a factory. Tune into a very natural way of thinking and wanting to be close to the earth, because we are a part of nature in its truest form. Take it further still, and marvel at how amazing our planet and all that it contains is! Consider that your food grows out of the soil and nourishes your body! Be grateful from your most authentic place that our world and bodies are absolutely incredible. This gratitude will not only dictate your attitude for the rest of the morning, but it will draw more to be grateful for.

Assignment:

What are 5 things that you are immediately grateful for?
1.
2.
3.
4.
5.

What are 5 things that you are grateful for in advance?
1.
2.
3.
4.
5.

What are 5 qualities that you really like about yourself?
1.
2.
3.
4.
5.

What are the qualities that are going to make you successful in your journey with wellness?

1.

2.

3.

4.

5.

Draw from what you've written above to create new thought patterns.

Routine

I highly encourage you to create rituals around your wellness. Rituals encourage consistency and consistency is what is going to bring you results. It's not enough to just really want to take control of your health, your actions must be consistent with your desire. At a very deep level, we have a strong need to stay consistent with how we define ourselves. Again, the words we speak over our lives, our health, our bodies really matter! If you define yourself in a negative way, perhaps believing at a deep level that you will never have control of your health, then your actions are going to be consistent with that belief. You will show again and again who you are at the deepest level. Empower yourself through creating rituals that ensure action is making your wishes a reality.

Morning is the natural time to begin a healthy routine. Our bodies are, hopefully, well rested, our stomachs are empty, and our minds are fresh. The quiet of the early morning is by far my favorite time to do a little yoga, pray, meditate and visualize. I also use this time to set my stomach up for success by drinking warm water with lemon before anything else enters my system. After breakfast I take my supplements and a spoonful of coconut oil before dropping the kids at school and leaving the house for the day.

Assignment:

What does your ideal morning look like?

What are 3 things that you can do right now to create room for a healthy morning routine?

Wellness can be almost a full-time job. Really though, what else is there? We absolutely must take care of ourselves so that we can live great lives and better love those around us. You are the only you there is and what you have to offer is something that no one else can. No one has your unique combination of gifts, perspective, personality and life experience. You matter!

In our fast-paced societies, we are too often disconnected from the wild, the natural and the organic world to which we actually belong. As you walk this journey, please do so with gratitude for how well designed all of this is. Rather than merely being okay with more fruits and vegetables, embrace them for all that they will do for your physical and mental wellbeing. Embrace them because life is beautiful, and your body is an amazing part of that! Embrace the beauty of living close to the Earth.

Habits

We all have them. Most are so innocuous one might be hard pressed to call them a habit. The way in which you mindlessly pick up your toothbrush and toothpaste in the morning, the angle you use to you squeeze the tube and place it back down in the exact same position and place that you do every day. The rhythm with which you tap your toothbrush against the sink when you are done. These are habits that help us quickly and efficiently move through our day.

Other habits are not so friendly, they pick us up like rag dolls, fling us around in the air, limbs flailing, drool flying, equilibrium a mass of confusion, and throw us every which direction as if we and our determination to change the habit were uncared for children's toys. These are the habits that set us back. These are the habits we're are burning to change yet seem to cling to desperately. These are the habits which reinforce the stories we believe about ourselves, the ones that are fiercely protecting the idea, true or false, of who we believe ourselves to be. Tuning into the stories and words we tell ourselves, owning our stories and recognizing what we have believed about ourselves, is a powerful tool in changing unwanted habits.

In his book, <u>The Power of Habit</u>, Charles Duhigg explains that habits help us conserve mental effort. We slip into the habit and therefore have less figuring out to do. That is why when you are on autopilot while brushing your teeth, you can mentally be reviewing your goals for the day. The habit of your motions and actions allows for your mind to go elsewhere.

Our habits include a cue, a routine and a reward. Certain times of day, emotions or events can act as cues which prompt us into the habit. According to Duhigg, in order to create a new habit, taking fish oil after breakfast for example, you must not only create a new cue, but you must create an obsession for the desired results. So, the cue is breakfast, the action is taking the fish oil and the desired result is lubrication for your joints, and moisture to your skin, hair and nails, decrease of inflammation and less popping and cracking as you move around through the day. There will be a point where you realize the fish oil is helping, but before then, it is up to you to become obsessed with the idea of nourishing your body with oil. Visualize and see the results, feel the results and become obsessed with the results. This is what is going to drive your new habit. According to Duhigg, your brain needs the anticipation of the reward in order to create the habit.

I talk about energy, how everything is made of it and how like energy draws like energy towards it. It's the Law of Attraction. When you are connecting emotionally with your desired result, you are pulling that energy toward you. Connect with the version of you you know needs to be played out. Connect with the fish oil popping, anti-inflammatory eating, healthy self that you know has always been inside. Visualize the oil coating your joints and connect with your desired results to the point that it is an obsession. This is a big help when you are trying to create new habits.

Assignment:

What is a habit you would like to develop?

What drives you to want to create this habit?

What will your cue be?

What will the reward be?

When you connect with it emotionally how do you feel?

Do you stand taller when you connect emotionally with your desired outcome?

How obsessed can you become with feeling this way?

Write out a scenario where you will be practicing your new habit. Write in detail how the cue, your actions and the reward take place.

Assignment:

What habit would you like to change?

Why would you like to change it?

Have you listened yet to your stories surrounding this habit? What story or belief about yourself are you reinforcing by continuing this habit?

Is the story or belief true?!
Dismantle the old, tired, no longer fitting idea....
Have you changed since you accepted that belief?
Is the belief keeping you small?

After dismantling the belief, replace it with the new and true story.
What are you replacing it with?

Can you connect emotionally to this version of you?

On a separate index card write your goal out along with the obsession that comes with it. Keep the card in a place where you will see it frequently. Read it multiple times a day and allow your subconscious to claim the new storyline.

Get Ready for Success

You are ready.
You are fully equipped to make this change.
Practically speaking, you have your shopping list, some meal plans and some amazing recipes. This however is not where the challenge dwells. The biggest challenge is in your mind. You know how to listen to your words and stories. You know how to replace negative thought patterns and you have a stated goal which is totally worth becoming excited over.
It's worth becoming obsessed over!
Become obsessed with your desired outcome. Become obsessed with our incredible world; with the interconnectedness of all the natural world and with how your health and vitality will increase once you harness your new knowledge as well as your amazing power to shape your reality.

YOU are in charge of your life.
YOU get to choose your path.

Become clear on your stories and what you believe about yourself.
Dissect, dethrone, and discard any old, hindering beliefs and replace them with new ones.

Focus on what you DO want.
Create your goal and become obsessed with it!

There is absolutely no reason why you shouldn't be able to do this. If there is, grab it, own it, dissect it and declare it untrue. You are strong and capable and in charge of your food choices as well as your attitude and your words. I know you can make this change just as I know that you deserve to feel good and make the most out of your life.

If you would like coaching, motivation, or encouragement, I am here for you. It's what I do best and I'm ready to walk with you on this journey.

Set up an appointment with me and let's answer any questions you have, tear down any obstacles that are in your way, reframe tired stories, and refine your action plan for success.

You can find me at Taproots805.com
Follow Taproots805 on Instagram and Facebook.

Recipes

Annie's Blueberry Kale Smoothie
2 cups Kale or Spinach or both
2-3 cups frozen Blueberries (as many as you can squeeze in there!)
2 Tbls Flaxseed
1/3 cup Cherry Juice
1 cup Almond Milk (or Coconut Milk)
Fill the rest w Water, Coconut Water, or Aloe Juice
Add Protein Powder, Turmeric and any other supplements.
Blend and Drink

THE BBP Smoothie (blueberry, beet and pineapple)
2 cups Kale or Spinach or both
1 cup frozen Blueberries
½ cup frozen beet chunks
½ cup fresh pineapple
2 Tbls Flaxseed
1/3 cup Cherry Juice
1 cup Almond Milk (or Coconut Milk)

Fill the rest w Water, Coconut Water, or Aloe Juice
Add Protein Powder, Turmeric and any other supplements.
Blend and Drink

Creamy Chocolate Hazelnut Shake with Chia (<u>48</u>)

3/4 cup water

1/4 cup whole hazelnuts (with or without skin), soaked overnight
and drained

1 tablespoon chia seeds

1 tablespoon raw cacao powder, or cocoa powder

3 to 4 dates, pitted

pinch of salt

10 ice cubes

Combine the water, hazelnuts, chia seeds, cacao powder, dates, and salt in a high-speed blender, and blend until smooth. Adjust any ingredients to taste, then add in the ice and blend again to create a milkshake-like texture.

Gwyneth Paltrow's Blueberry Cauliflower Smoothie

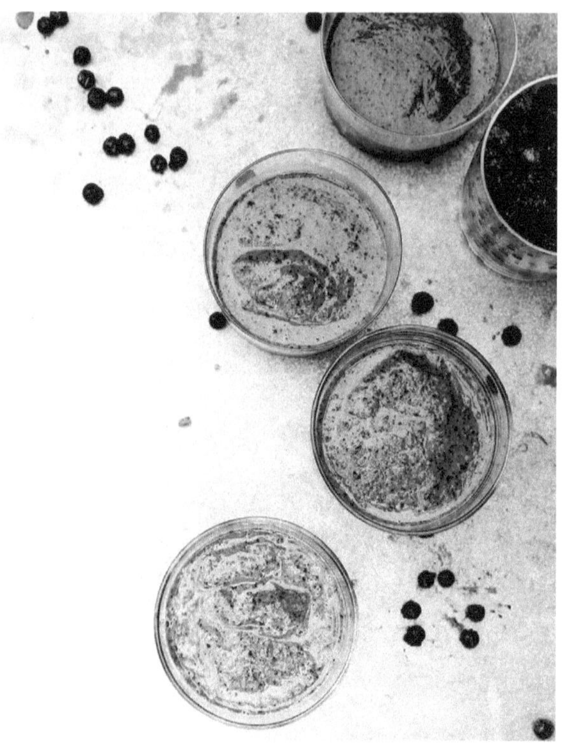

½ cup frozen blueberries

½ cup frozen cauliflower

1 tablespoon unsweetened almond butter

¾ cup unsweetened almond milk

1 date, pitted and roughly chopped

Juice of ½ lime

Blend and enjoy.

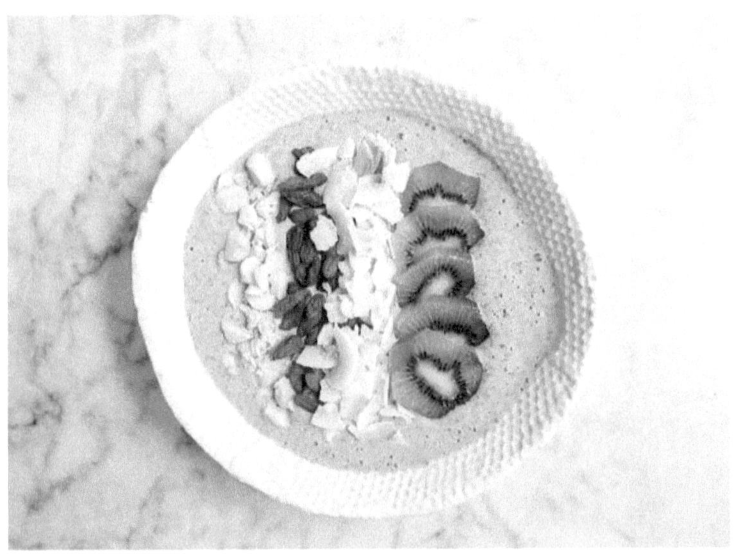

PHOTO: LIZ ANDREW/STYLING: ERIN MCDOWELL

GREEN SMOOTHIE BOWL

1 frozen banana

1 avocado

2 cups spinach

1 apple

¼ cup almond milk

½ cup ice

blend until smooth. Pour the smoothie into a bowl and garnish with 2 tablespoons goji berries, 2 tablespoons toasted coconut, 1 tablespoon chopped macadamia nuts and 1 sliced kiwi or whatever beautiful combination of fruit, nuts and berries your heart desires.

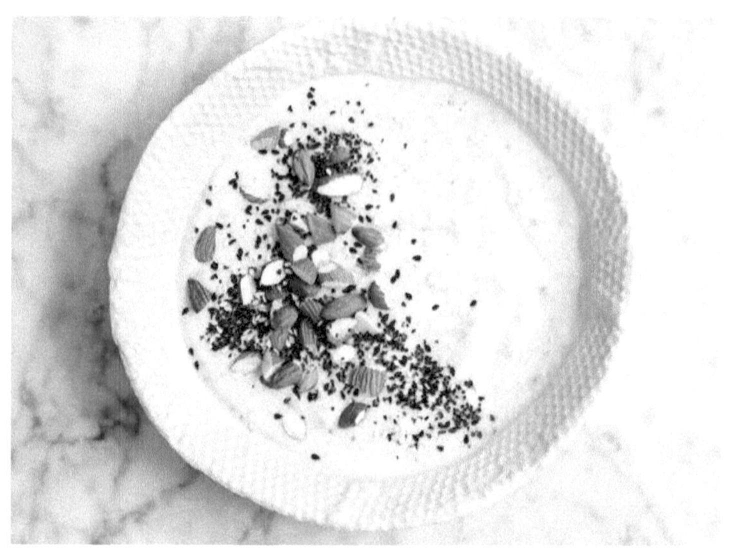

PHOTO: LIZ ANDREW/STYLING: ERIN MCDOWELL

VANILLA-OAT SMOOTHIE BOWL

1 frozen banana

1/3 cup Greek yogurt

¼ cup almond milk

1/3 cup rolled oats

1 teaspoon honey

¼ teaspoon pure vanilla extract

a pinch of ground cinnamon

½ cup ice

blend until smooth. Pour the smoothie into a bowl and garnish with ¼ cup chopped almonds, 2 tablespoons cocoa nibs and 2 tablespoons sesame seeds.

Overnight Oats

2 cups gluten-free Rolled Oats
2 cups Almond Milk or any other milk of choice

Mix the oats and the milk together in a bowl, cover and let sit in the refrigerator overnight. The oats will soak up the liquid and become tender by morning. However, just oats and milk is a little plain, so...

think about adding in:
Berries or other fruit
Cinnamon
Seeds
Honey
Maple Syrup
Nut butter
Vanilla

Morning Custard

½ cup Blueberries
½ cup Shredded Coconut
3 tbls Chia Seeds
2 tbls plain yogurt

Ground cinnamon to taste
Almond Milk (or any other milk)

Combine the berries, coconut and chia seeds and cinnamon in a bowl. Cover the mixture with milk. The more milk you use, the thinner the custard will be in the morning. Cover and let sit in the refrigerator overnight. This recipe works great with any fruit and with a wide variety of add ins. Be creative. The key is to have the chia seeds and plenty of liquid for them to absorb.

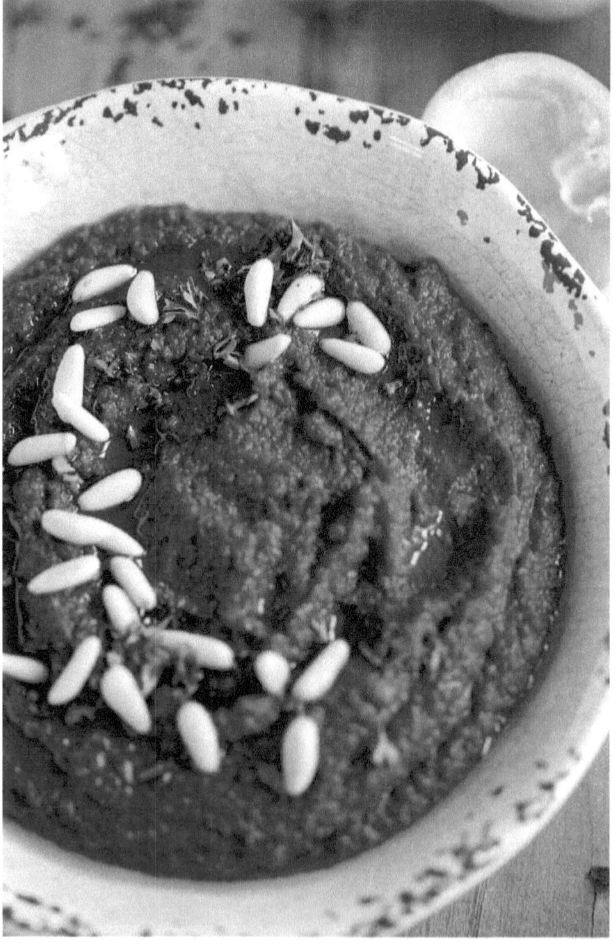

Beetroot and lemon hummus (50)

6 medium size beetroots (either ready-cooked from the supermarket, or you can roast and peel your own)

A 400g tin of ready-cooked chickpeas (about 2 American cups in size)

1 tablespoon of tahini (a paste made from sesame seeds and usually found in the "World" aisle or "Free From" sections of supermarkets)

The juice of 2 lemons, squeezed
5 tablespoons of extra virgin olive oil
Half a teaspoon of sea salt flakes
A pinch of ground pepper

Put all the ingredients in a powerful blender and pulse till smooth.
Spoon out into a bowl and spread the hummus on bread, warm toast for breakfast, or used as a dip for crunchy vegetables such as celery, carrots, radishes - you choose!
Can be kept in the fridge for 2-3 days.

Easy Homemade Lentil Hummus

1 15-ounce can lentils, rinsed and drained
1/2 cup sesame tahini
1 clove garlic, peeled and smashed
1/4 cup extra virgin olive oil
3 tablespoons freshly squeezed lemon juice
1/2 teaspoon salt
1/2 teaspoon ground cumin
1/4 cup water

Mix all ingredients except water in a food processor on high speed until very finely chopped.

Scrape the sides of the bowl down with a rubber spatula, add water, and process again until smooth.

Serve immediately, or store in the refrigerator in an airtight container up to one week.

– Jess Thomson, graduate of The Cambridge School of Culinary Arts, awarded the certified culinary professional (CCP) designation by the International Association of Culinary Professionals.

Red Thai Curry

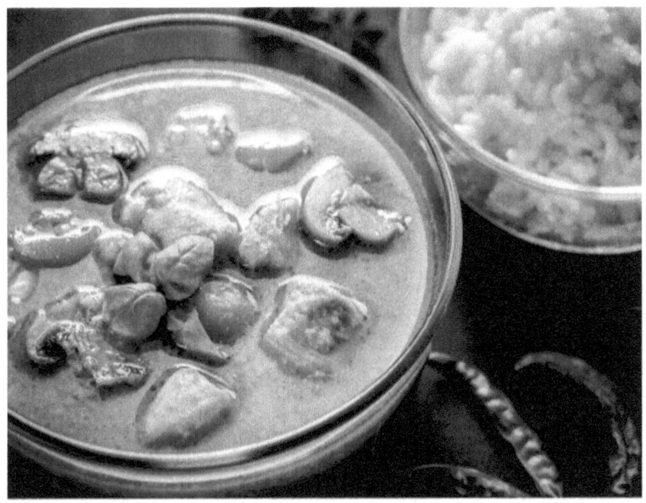

This recipe is courtesy of Dr. Weil's cookbook: FAST FOOD GOOD FOOD.

2 tablespoons grapeseed oil

1 tablespoon minced peeled ginger

3 garlic cloves, pressed and allowed to sit for 10 minutes

1 1/2 tablespoons Thai red curry paste

2 carrots, peeled and sliced on the bias

1 small Yukon gold potato, diced into 1/2-inch cubes

1 red bell pepper, seeded and diced into 1/2-inch pieces

2 (16-ounce) cans light coconut milk

2 tablespoons fish sauce

1 pound broccoli florets

8 ounces extra-firm tofu, cut into 3/4-inch cubes

2 teaspoons grated lime zest

1 tablespoon lime juice

1/2 teaspoon grade B maple syrup

4 scallions, white and light green parts only, thinly sliced on the bias

1/4 cup packed fresh cilantro leaves, coarsely chopped

Lime wedges

1. Heat the oil in a large wide pan over medium heat. Add the ginger, garlic, and red curry paste, cook for 45 seconds, then add the carrots and sauté for 3 minutes.
2. Add the potatoes and peppers, stir to coat, and sauté for 2 minutes. Stir in the coconut milk, 1 cup of water, and the fish sauce and bring to a simmer. Cook, stirring occasionally, until the liquid is thickened and slightly reduced, and the potatoes are just tender, about 8 minutes. Add the broccoli and tofu and cook, covered, until the broccoli is crisp-tender, and the tofu is heated through, about 2 minutes.
3. Remove from the heat and stir in the lime zest, lime juice, and maple syrup. Top each portion with scallions, chopped cilantro, and a lime wedge.

Spiced Diver Scallops

¼ cup toasted almonds
½ teaspoon sea salt
¼ teaspoon lemongrass powder
⅛ teaspoon togarashi pepper mix
10 fennel seeds
18 scallops, U-10 size, extra large
2 tablespoon chopped fresh parsley
2 tablespoons extra virgin olive oil

In a spice grinder, pulverize almonds, salt, lemongrass powder, togarashi pepper mix and fennel seeds.
In a large bowl, toss scallops with spice mix and parsley.

Heat the olive oil in a large, nonstick skillet over high heat. Add half the scallops. Cook 1 minute. Turn. Cook additional 1 minute, or until done. Remove scallops from pan and set aside. Cook the remaining scallops.

Blistered Green Beans with Tomatoes, Pounded Walnuts and Squash (<u>50</u>)

1 cup walnuts, toasted
½ bunch parsley, roughly chopped
Zest and juice of 1 lemon
¼ cup olive oil
Kosher salt
1 tablespoon neutral oil, like canola
1-pound green beans, stems snapped off
1-pint cherry tomatoes, halved
1 medium summer squash, shaved into paper-thin planks or rounds

Place the walnuts in a clean cloth or towel. You need to make sure the ends are closed, then bash the walnuts with the bottom of a frying pan until they are in pieces and have released some oil. It's an easy alternative to wasting plastic and putting even more of it into our Earth.

Combine the walnuts, parsley, lemon zest and juice, olive oil and a pinch of salt, and stir to combine.

Heat the neutral oil until smoking hot and add the green beans with a pinch of salt. Let the green beans blister, then toss to coat, flip and blister the other side.

Remove from the heat and toss with the tomatoes and summer squash. Top with the walnut mixture and serve.

Cauliflower Pizza Dough (51)

1 head cauliflower, stalk removed
1/2 cup shredded mozzarella
1/4 cup grated Parmesan
1/2 teaspoon dried oregano
1/2 teaspoon kosher salt
1/4 teaspoon garlic powder
2 eggs, lightly beaten

Preheat the oven to 400 degrees F.

Line a baking sheet with parchment paper.

Break the cauliflower into florets and pulse in a food processor until fine.

Steam in a steamer basket and drain well.

Let cool.

In a bowl, combine the cauliflower with the mozzarella, Parmesan, oregano, salt, garlic powder and eggs. Transfer to the center of the baking sheet and spread into a circle, resembling a pizza crust. Bake for 20 minutes.

Add desired toppings and bake an additional 10 minutes

Ecuadorian Tabbouleh

2 cups quinoa
4 cups water
¼ cup chopped red onion
½ cup chopped cilantro
½ cup chopped fresh mint
½ cup chopped fresh parsley
$1/3$ cup extra virgin olive oil
2 tablespoon lemon juice
3 tablespoons fresh lime juice
1 avocado, peeled, pitted and diced
4 tomatoes, peeled, seeded and diced
2 pepino melons, peeled, seeded and diced
Sea salt and freshly ground black pepper

Wash the quinoa under running water. Place in medium pan. Add the water and bring to boil. Reduce heat to low. Cover and simmer until liquid is absorbed, approximately 10-15 minutes.

Remove from heat; quinoa will be somewhat translucent. Fluff with fork, and transfer quinoa to large bowl. Let cool to room temperature.

In a mixing bowl combine red onion, cilantro, mint, parsley, olive oil, lemon and lime juices.

Add avocado, tomatoes and melon.

Add mixture to quinoa. Toss gently. Season to taste with salt and pepper.

Chipotle Black Bean Soup

1 Yellow onion
2 Tsp. olive oil
1 clove garlic
12 cup carrots
Chicken or vegetable broth
Chipotle Chili Powder

Sauté 1/2 small yellow onion (chopped) in 2 tsp. olive oil over medium-low heat until soft.

Add beans, 1 smashed garlic clove, 2 cups chicken or vegetable broth, 1/4 to 1/2 tsp. chipotle chili powder (to taste) and a handful of baby carrots.

Simmer 10 minutes, or until carrots are soft, and then puree.

Season with salt and pepper.

Spinach Salad with Strawberry–Poppy Seed Vinaigrette

1 16 oz. container strawberries (about 20 large), tops removed
1 small shallot, finely chopped
2 Tbs. apple cider vinegar
1/2 tsp. salt
Freshly ground pepper
1/4 cup extra virgin olive oil
1 Tbs. poppy seeds
4 ounces baby spinach (about 4 big handfuls)
1/2 cup crumbled feta cheese

3/4 cup chopped walnuts
1/4 cup pickled red onions (recipe follows), optional

Slice half the strawberries and set them aside for the spinach salad. Remove the hulls from the remaining berries so that only the red parts remain, and coarsely chop.

Place the chopped strawberries, shallots, vinegar, salt and a few grindings of pepper in a blender, and blend on high until smooth. Add the oil and poppy seeds, and blend again. Season to taste with salt and pepper if needed and transfer to a serving container.

Place the spinach, feta, walnuts, onions and reserved strawberries in a large bowl. Add strawberry–poppy seed vinaigrette (to taste) and toss the spinach salad just before serving.

Seeded Rice

1 cup whole grain rice
¼ cup raw pumpkin seeds, sunflower seeds or a combination
2 ¼ cup water or low-sodium vegetable broth
½ teaspoon salt

Rinse rice and drain in colander or sieve.
 Place in large bowl and cover with water. Soak overnight.
Throw off the soaking water.

In a pot with tight-fitting lid, combine rice, seeds, water or broth and salt.

Cook over high heat until boiling, then reduce to low and simmer 45 to 50 minutes. Remove pot from heat and let sit 5 to 10 minutes, then fluff with wooden spoon.

Note: this recipe is excerpted from The Healthiest Meals on Earth by Jonny Bowden, PhD

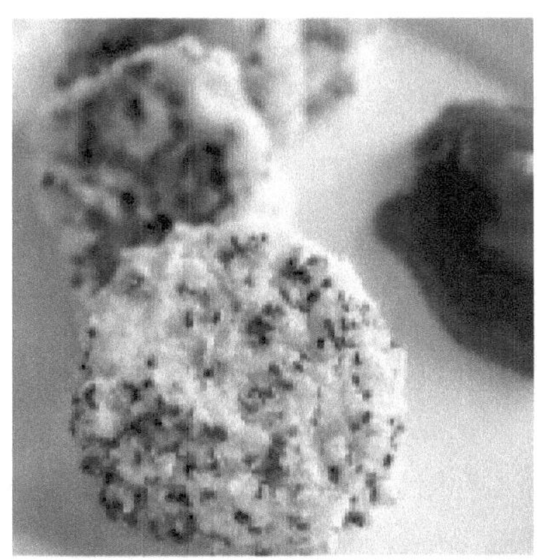

Cauliflower Medallions- Lisa Lin

1/2 head of cauliflower, florets only

1 large egg

1 large egg white

1/2 cup mozzarella

1/2 cup onions, diced

1/4 cup parsley, chopped

3 tbls almond meal

2 tbls organic cornmeal

2 tbls chia seeds

salt and pepper, to taste

dried herbs (optional)

Preheat oven to 400 degrees F. Grease two cookie sheets.

Fill a saucepan up with 2 to 3 inches of water and bring it to boil. Once the water is boiled, place the cauliflower florets in the saucepan. Cook for about 5 minutes. Drain the boiled water from the saucepan and run the cauliflower under cold water.

Put the cauliflower, cheese, onions, and parsley in a food processor and mix until everything is finely chopped.

Empty the cauliflower mixture into a bowl and stir in the egg and egg white.

Add the almond meal, corn meal, chia seeds, salt, pepper, and any dried herbs, and fold everything into the cauliflower mixture.

Scoop about a tablespoon of the mixture and place it on the cookie sheet. Flatten the mixture into small medallions.

Once all the mixture is placed on the cookie sheets, place the sheets into the oven.

Bake for about 16 to 20 minutes and flip the medallions halfway through the baking.

Remove the medallions from the oven when they are golden brown.

Makes 30 to 35 Medallions

Chia Chipotle Dressing- Terry Hope Romero

1/2 cup freshly squeezed or store-bought orange juice
3 tablespoons freshly squeezed lime juice
2 tablespoons olive oil
1 tablespoon chopped chipotle chiles in adobo sauce
2 teaspoons agave nectar
1 tablespoon chia seeds
1 clove garlic, minced
1/2 teaspoon ground cumin
1/2 teaspoon salt

Whisk together all of the ingredients in a glass or plastic measuring cup. Cover and chill for 10 minutes or overnight to plump up the chia seeds. Store chilled and use within 2 days for best flavor.

Dr. Axe's ACV Tonic (47)

1 glass of warm or hot water
2 Tbsp apple cider vinegar
1/2 lemon, juiced
½ tsp of fresh ground ginger
1 dash cayenne pepper or cinnamon
1 tsp raw, local honey (optional)
Warm the water. Mix all ingredients together (adding honey makes it more palatable for those new to ACV). Drink warm.

Turmeric Tea

Bring four cups of water to a boil.
Add one teaspoon of ground turmeric and reduce to a simmer for 10 minutes.
Strain the tea through a fine sieve into a cup; add honey and/or lemon to taste.
Add a pinch of black pepper to increase absorption.

Pickled Grapes- Jessica Goldman

5 to 6 handfuls of seedless black or red grapes
2 teaspoons of yellow mustard seed
1 cinnamon stick

2 cups of white wine or champagne vinegar
1 teaspoon of black peppercorn

Pick up some plump, seedless black or red grapes and slice off the belly buttons (the top part where the stem was) of five or six handfuls. By taking off this top piece of the grape, you will allow the pickling juices to seep into the fruit immediately.

Fill a small Mason jar with the grapes, 2 teaspoons of yellow mustard seed, and one stick of cinnamon. Or, as in my case, use 3 teaspoons of ground cinnamon if you forget to buy cinnamon sticks.

Heat two cups of white wine or champagne vinegar in a pot with 1 teaspoon of black peppercorns. Remove from heat once it boils.

Let the pickling liquid (step 3) fully cool before filling the Mason jar. This will keep the fruit from becoming too mushy.

Shake and shimmy your Mason jar and put in refrigerator. The grapes will be pickled in two days.

References

1. Healthlihttps://www.healthline.com/nutrition/is-leaky-gut-realne.com- Is Leaky Gut Syndrome a Real condition? An Unbias Look, Becky Belll MS, RD
2. https://www.frontiersin.org/journals/immunology/sections/inflammation
3. Wheat Belly- Dr. William Davis
4. Wheat Belly; Total Health- Dr. William Davis
5. https://www.amazon.com/Hidden-Life-Trees-Communicate_Discoveries-Secret/dp/1771642483
6. https://yurielkaim.com/wheat-free-diet/
7. Sources: Sweet little Lies, The Bitter Truth About Sugar- Christopher Delattore
8. https://www.cdc.gov/nutrition/index.html
9. RayandTerry.com/wellness_information
10. Elev8.com/six-foods-that-contain-hidden-sugar
11. womenshealthmag.com/food/g19990590/sugar-facts
12. Nutribullet- Pocket Nutrition- Nutrition Guide
13. https://www.louisehay.com/18-amazing-health-benefits-bone-broth/
14. https://draxe.com/boswellia/

15. https://draxe.com/bromelain/

16. https://nccih.nih.gov/health/glucosaminechondroitin

17. https://www.healthline.com/nutrition/11-proven-benefits-of-ginger#section1

18. https://draxe.com/msm-supplement/

19. https://www.healthline.com/nutrition/17-health-benefits-of-omega-3#section8

20. https://www.medicalnewstoday.com/articles/161618.php

21. https://www.health.harvard.edu/vitamins-and-supplements/health-benefits-of-taking-probiotics

22. https://www.prebiotin.com/prebiotin-academy/what-are-prebiotics/prebiotics-vs-probiotics/

23. https://draxe.com/what-is-collagen/

24. https://www.verywellhealth.com/hyaluronic-acid-supplements-89465

25. https://www.healthline.com/nutrition/hyaluronic-acid-benefits#section6

26. https://www.arthritis.org/living-with-arthritis/treatments/natural/supplements-herbs/guide/glucosamine.php

27. https://www.healthline.com/nutrition/glucosamine#other-uses

28. http://www.whfoods.com/genpage.php?tname=foodspice&dbid=78

29. https://www.healthline.com/nutrition/why-is-fiber-good-for-you#section7

30. https://draxe.com/slippery-elm/

31. You are a Badass: How to Stop Doubting Your Greatness and Start Living an Awesome Life- Jen Sincero

32. https://aaptiv.com/magazine/gut-health-tips

33. https://www.ncbi.nlm.nih.gov/pmc/articles/PMC4991899/ https://www.ncbi.nlm.nih.gov/pubmed/20203603

34. https://www.healthline.com/nutrition/ gut-microbiome-and-health#section1

35. https://hummkombucha.com/the-difference-betwee n-good-bacteria-and-bad-bacteria/

36. https://www.medicalnewstoday.com/articles/323214.php

37. https://www.healthline.com/ nutrition/19-best-prebiotic-foods#section13

38. https://draxe.com/probiotic-foods/

39. https://www.mindbodygreen.com/0-9331/top-10-probioti c-foods-to-add-to-your-diet.html

40. https://www.healthline.com/ nutrition/12-benefits-of-meditation#section4

41. https://www.scienceofpeople.com/meditation-benefits/

42. https://www.psychologytoday.com/us/blog/feeling-it/201 309/20-scientific-reasons-start-meditating-today

43. https://ghr.nlm.nih.gov/condition/ lactose-intolerance#statistics

44. https://www.mindbodygreen.com/0-8646/ the-dangers-of-dairy.html

45. Ht

46. tps://system.na3.netsuite.com/core/media/media.nl?id=67 145&c=460947&h=77a950d2ff4031c51502&_xt=.pdf

47. https://8fit.com/nutrition/apple-cider-vinegar-myth s-truths-and-ways-to-use-it/

48. https://detoxinista.com/creamy-chocolate-hazelnut-shak e-vegan-paleo/

49. http://www.jeannettehyde.com/healthy-recipes.htm

50. https://www.purewow.com/recipes/
blistered-green-beans-walnuts-squash

51. https://www.foodnetwork.com/recipes/katie-lee/
cauliflower-pizza-crust-2651381

52. https://www.healthline.com/nutrition/benefits-of-cloves

53. https://www.psychologytoday.
com/us/blog/flourish/200912/
seeing-is-believing-the-power-visualization

54. https://entrepreneurs.maqtoob.com/4-scientifi
c-reasons-why-visualization-will-increa
se-your-chances-to-succeed-5515ef2dbdb7

55. https://www.healthline.com/nutrition/
fruit-juice-is-just-as-bad-as-soda#section3

56. https://www.cnn.com/2019/05/17/health/fruit-juice-sugar
y-drink-early-death-study/index.html

57. https://www.ncbi.nlm.nih.gov/pmc/articles/PMC3815616/

58. https://entrepreneurs.maqtoob.com/4-scientifi
c-reasons-why-visualization-will-increa
se-your-chances-to-succeed-5515ef2dbdb7

59. https://thewellnessenterprise.com/emoto/#top

60. https://www.intuitiveeating.
org/10-principles-of-intuitive-eating/

61. https://www.livescience.com/52344-inflammation.html

62. https://www.health.harvard.edu/newsletter_article/
Inflammation_A_unifying_theory_of_disease

63. https://www.medicalmedium.com/
medical-medium-celery-juice-movement.htm

www.ingramcontent.com/pod-product-compliance
Lightning Source LLC
Chambersburg PA
CBHW031231250726
48655CB00005B/1906